Gifts of Love and Life

Best wishes to
Stella,
a lovely friend whom
I have had the pleasure
of meeting.
With love,
Helen Nazarian Pompeian
28 September 2006

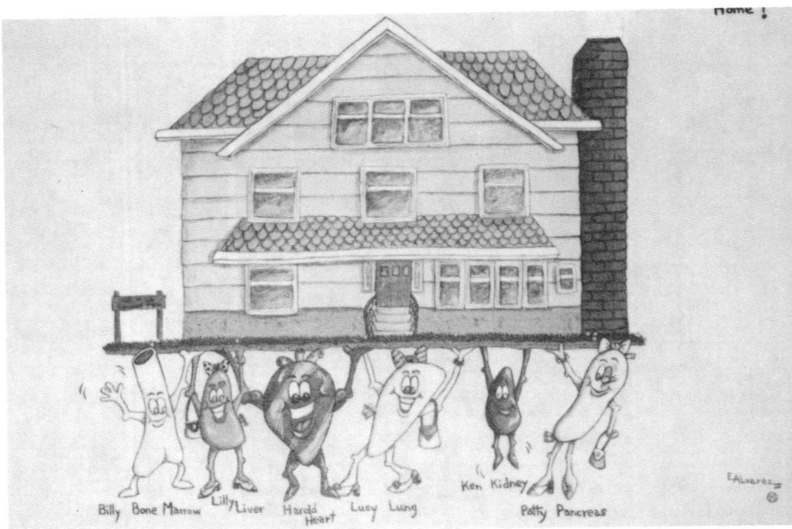

Transplant Organs: Concept of Edward Alvarez created during his mother's residency at Gift of Life Transplant House. Left to right: Billy Bone Marrow, Lilly Liver, Harold Heart, Lucy Lung, Ken Kidney, and Patty Pancreas.

Gifts of Love and Life

Helen Nazarian Pompeian

VANTAGE PRESS
New York

FIRST EDITION

Published by Vantage Press, Inc.
516 West 34th Street, New York, New York 10001

Manufactured in the United States of America
ISBN: 0-533-11454-3

Library of Congress Catalog Card No.: 95-90064

0 9 8 7 6 5 4 3

To all those dearest to me:
my son, Edward,
his wife, Jayne,
my daughter, Sharon,
and all my beloved grandchildren:
Paul, Edward, Aaron, Nicholas, and Adrienne,
and my mother and brothers and sisters.

Contents

Foreword

The early days of my brother Edward's long and serious illness were unreal to me, a teenager. My father, mother, brother, and I were a happy and healthy family. In my limited knowledge of illness and unhappiness, my close-by relatives, including my grandmother, were happy and healthy.

Of course, as all youngsters do, Edward and I suffered skinned knees, bumps and bruises, and other mishaps that hurt. We cried. Mother or Grandmother, always on hand, administered appropriate first aid, applied some healing lotion, probably added a Band-Aid or bandage, wiped away the tears, and ended the process with a hug and kiss. In a short time the hurt was forgotten, and we were healed. We had chicken pox and measles, bites and rashes, and colds to make us miserable. But Mother or Grandmother nursed us quickly back to good health.

So, what was this terrible thing that happened to my little brother? This something that changed every aspect of our lives, what was it? We were no longer a happy, healthy, carefree family. It took me a long, long time to even begin to realize the seriousness of a debilitating illness and its effect on a loving family.

My little brother was examined by many doctors and underwent many tests in a number of hospitals, but no absolute diagnosis was made. There continued to be manifestations of new complications. Medication in variety and quantity that was unbelievable was administered, and his condition continued to worsen.

The toll on our mother became a real concern for us. She was sick with worry, exhausted by so many hours in the hospitals and disturbed sleep, brokenhearted watching her beloved son losing his strength and stamina, and terrified because there seemed so little or no help.

The miracle happened when we finally made arrangements for my brother to be examined at the Mayo Clinic, Rochester, Minnesota. There, at that great medical institution, we were given reason to believe that he really would recover. And we, the family, learned about marvels of medical skill and knowledge. His recovery took a very long time—years—but we knew he was recovering.

Much later, I suggested to Mother that she write a book. Her experiences and Edward's were filled with pain and misery, trials and tribulations, frustrations and endurance, worry and fear, despair and hope. We believed in the power of prayer, but many times it seemed that our prayers were not heard.

It took months and years, such a long time, but looking back, we began to understand that Edward had steadfastly held onto the gift of life through countless miracles.

Here is a true and remarkable human interest story, a story to offer hope and encouragement to those who are suffering similar circumstances.

These few words were written affectionately for my mother's book.

—Sharon

Acknowledgments

I extend my warm thanks and gratitude to many friends and members of my family who gave me their helpful encouragement and kind support. I am especially grateful to Dr. Carl F. Anderson, Dr. William J. Johnson, and Dr. John E. Woods of the Mayo Clinic for their time and talent on my behalf; to Mrs. Eleonore Clappier, who did far more than edit the book; to my nephew; Earl P. Cook, who added valuable suggestions for the book; to Edward Alvarez, whose painting, the frontispiece of this book, is a clever concept of organs for transplantation; and to my eleven-year-old grandson, Edward Paul, for his fine drawing of the new Gift of Life Transplant house; to Sr. Margeen Hoffmann, OFS, Executive Director of the new home, who was very helpful to me in many ways; and to Sr. Jane Frances Gregoire, OFS, Facilities Manager.

Drs. John E. Woods and Frank J. Leary performed most of the original surgery. These operations included removal of Edward's kidneys, appendix, and spleen, the removal of the donor kidney, and its transplantation into Edward.

Many other surgeons and physicians were involved in Edward's care: Drs. E. C. Burke, Peter Frohnert, Artin Jibilian, S. B. Kurtz, J. C. Mitchell, H. O. Perry, F. H. Sim, Sylvester Sterioff, J. A. Velosa, W. R. Wagoner, Horst Zincke, Mr. J. J. Chihak, and so many others beyond my ability to mention.

Through countless years these dear and kind people have given me strength, consolation and comfort—Zabel

(Melkonian) Allison, Mr. and Mrs. Nazar Hajinian, cousin Agnes Melkonian, Marion L. Steeber, and Rose Soditch. I give them my heartfelt thanks for all they have done to support me through all my years of worry and pain.

Prologue

This book, part biography and part autobiography, focuses on the impact a serious illness, my son's, has had on our family's lives and the lives of others. My story, and I think I can rightly call it a story, began when my son, Edward, was eleven years old. His sister, Sharon, is older by five years. He was born on November 26, 1951, and his loving and devoted sister made herself his little mother.

We were a family raised in the tradition of Armenian culture, with its bearing on the home. The husband was the head of the household and the absolute authoritarian. The wife was the keeper of the home and children and helpmate of the husband. She was expected to be in agreement with him always. We had a nice home in a small city in Michigan, close to many relatives, and I enjoyed keeping it orderly and attractive. I made every effort to please my husband both at home and sometimes helping at his place of business. Also, I did secretarial work for many years. My mother, who lived near us, was happy to take care of the children when I was away from them at work. I loved them beyond words. I knew my greatest pleasure when I could be at home with them, for the joy and fun they gave me. Watching them grow out of babyhood and develop their own unique personalities was a fascinating experience for me. I never forgot to count God's blessings for the precious gifts that my son and daughter were to me.

Sharon was an excellent student and always had

many friends, who remained close through thick and thin. They would enjoy themselves at each other's various homes doing whatever the moods of the day required. Sharon was a very capable and dependable little girl.

Edward found school a wonderful place. From the beginning he was a superior student, according to his teachers. He truly loved school, all his classmates, and his teachers. They, in turn, regarded him with warm affection. He loved to sing, and he liked to have me play the piano to accompany him. He learned many of the old songs as well as many of the current popular songs, and, having mastered whistling, he whistled the songs on the way home from school day after day. When I had reasonably completed my homely chores, I often would sit on our porch to enjoy his happy approach. He was a good mimic and did very well in his imitations of TV and other characters.

His birthday parties, until he was eleven years old, were special events, believe me. Everyone in Edward's class was invited and attended. It was a joy to see all of them coming down the street with Edward after school. To any suggestion of mine that we invite just a few, he would exclaim, "Oh, Mom, we can't do that! I want all of them, please!"

Was I living in a fantasy world of joy? I was young, not very mature, inexperienced, and unworldly. It never occurred to me that our lives would not continue in our own happy fashion. Who would ever think that our lovable, hale and hearty young boy was doomed to a frightful illness that would be life-threatening for years? Nothing in our lives or the experiences of any of our relatives could in any way prepare us for the agony of the endless years of critical illness suffered by our child from his eleventh year until he was well into adulthood.

My story goes on, somberly enough, with years of misdiagnosis and mismanagement of Edward's illness. This phase is epitomized by one doctor's cold and cruel statement to me: "Your son will not live to be sixteen." That was in the 1960s.

Through days and nights, watching at Edward's bedside in one hospital after another and at home, I had to do something—something quiet. I read, crocheted, looked through windows, and wrote letters. After a time I found myself writing notes about Edward's condition, his care and treatment. I found that this was the occupation best suited to my situation and my trying to keep in touch and gather some understanding of the fearful illness he was suffering. But how could I develop any understanding of an illness that seemed to defy diagnosis?

Since that time, Edward, though never entirely free of pain or other medical problems, has managed several years of college, established his own business, and raised a thriving family.

The turnabout in our lives came when a concerned couple recommended that we go to the Mayo Clinic in Rochester, Minnesota, for a reassessment of my son's condition. We did so, and in due time a definitive diagnosis was made—one kidney was found to be totally nonfunctioning and the other functioning only partially—and treatment was started. Several operations were needed, followed by years of treatment to build up Edward's strength. Then in April 1973, he received a kidney transplant, for which I was the donor.

Over the years of his illness, my son met and made friends with many people who themselves needed organ transplants. He also met their families, and having seen the toll his own experience had on his own family, he was moved to compassion for them as well. Organ transplant has indeed been a gift of life for Edward, and in his case, the experience inspired a dream, eventually realized, of establishing a "Gift of Life Transplant House" in support of transplant patients and their families. As soon as he was able, he strove to establish such a place, which would offer these people low-cost housing, kitchen, dining, and sleeping areas, and an opportunity to share with one another the good and bad days. Working tirelessly, he raised the initial $15,000 needed to make a down payment on a three-story house in Rochester that became the Gift of Life Transplant House. It opened to its first guests in 1984. Now, over ten years later, a much more spacious residence is being remodeled for the same purpose. It is expected to open in the summer of 1995.

My book is by no means a litany of clinical details. We have touched the lives of many and have been touched by them. These relationships are a rich source of additional anecdotes.

I believe that the total story that has emerged will speak to many, physically disadvantaged or not, because of what it says about what the challenged human spirit can achieve.

Long ago Sharon suggested that all my notes had the makings of a book. This was a far-out thought for me. Many years passed until I really began to wonder if I should try such a venture. I recognized that I had a message for famlies who are carrying the same burdens of worry, pain, and fear that my family had endured. I began to believe that an account of the wonderful recovery made by my son might inspire some confidence in others to at least wonder if miracles really can happen.

Gifts of Love and Life

CHAPTER I
The Beginning

What is a nightmare? Almost everyone knows it is a frightening and haunting dream, and many of us know that, in our conscious lives, there are nightmares. My family's nightmare, which lasted for years, began in the summer of 1963, with the onset of illness in our young son, Edward.

We lived very comfortably and most uneventfully in Pontiac, Michigan, in an area of well-kept homes, lovely lawns, and pleasant, friendly neighbors. A widow with no children who lived across the street from our home found the fun and games of our children and their friends a particularly enjoyable attraction when she was lonely. Our children, Sharon, a beautiful little girl, and Edward, a lively and lovable boy, were our greatest joy and great pleasure. We were very, very proud of them. They loved each other dearly, and there was no sibling jealousy between them. They considered themselves caretakers of each other. Loving relatives lived only a few miles away from us. We had many good times together—picnics, Sunday dinners, and holiday festivities.

Our children led a happy life, which they shared with their many friends. Edward, Ed or Eddie to his playmates, always kept his friends. God had blessed him with special qualities, a loving heart, a trusting soul and unlimited generosity. He really loved going to school, and he enjoyed and respected his teachers.

My mother, my sister Janet, my children, and I observed a little monthly social outing. I drove about twenty-five miles to Detroit, where we first visited our favorite store for shopping and then had lunch. Edward always enjoyed the time because he had the fun of choosing a new toy or game or book. Our first knowledge of his illness, and we had no way of knowing that this was the beginning of years of misery, happened during such an outing. We were just ready to have lunch when suddenly he complained of feeling sick. He started vomiting.

I called our family doctor and described as well as I could Edward's condition. The doctor advised me to take my son directly to his office. By the time we reached the doctor's office, Edward's illness had taken on new aspects. Answering the doctor's questioning, I agreed that Edward had been gaining weight for some time. It had never occurred to me that this could be a symptom of any illness.

After the examination, the doctor did not give us a diagnosis. He gave us a prescription for sulfa and told us to take Edward home. The sulfa, he said, should diminish the discomfort and lower Edward's temperature to normal, but he did not recover as we expected. He didn't regain much energy.

Several weeks later he became very sick again. The doctor told us to bring Edward to the hospital emergency room. From there he was taken to a hospital bed. After many tests, the tentative diagnoses included strep throat, pneumonia, and, it was assumed, he had a treatable form of kidney disease referred to as lupus nephritis. For this he was given high doses of steroids and chloroquine.

A very special blessing came to us at this hospital. Sam and Mary Leto came into our lives. Mary was a patient also and recovering well enough to visit Edward.

Sam spent time with Edward many, many times, and they became good friends. Sam told Edward about the Mayo Clinic and all the good that was done there for him and for people who had serious illnesses. Sam, a devout Catholic, told Edward about Padre Pio, a saintly priest in Italy who was renowned for his great healing powers. Sam had received from the padre several blessed medals that he had worn, joined together with a ribbon, on his various hospital gowns. He had strong feelings that wearing them and prayers would help him to recovery. He did experience an excellent recovery. He gave his medals to Edward to wear on his hospital gowns with prayers that he would regain his health. Sam also suggested that Edward, when he felt strong enough, write a letter to Padre Pio asking for his intervention to God that his health be restored. Edward wrote the letter, and Sam mailed it. In a relatively short time, Edward received a response and assurance that Padre Pio would indeed remember him in his prayers. Enclosed also was a small picture. Edward carried this picture on his person for many years and always believed that Padre Pio was helping him.

I wish I could really describe the wonderful support these two dear people, Mary and Sam, gave us with their love, help, and advice. Many times later I suffered deep regret that their advice at that time made so little impact on my thinking. I was so fatigued and distraught that their suggestions that I seek out better care for Edward fell on deaf ears.

When Edward, with a frightening accumulation of body fluid, was dismissed from the hospital in about two weeks, we had little to give us courage. Mary and Sam continued to give us the strength we needed to carry on.

After two weeks Edward's condition took on a new

and alarming change. He suffered a fearful accumulation of body fluid, which caused his whole abdominal area to be distended so that I thought he would burst. I asked his attending physician about the wisdom of having Edward examined elsewhere. He said, "I know of no other place. If I did, I would tell you." It is very hard to understand why my son's condition was dismissed so lightly at such a time.

We had no way of knowing that a very dark path was ahead of us. We refused to give up hope that our child would be healed. We somehow kept the faith and believed that our prayers would sometime bring us to the end of our sorrow and pain.

Home from the hospital, our son wanted to return to junior high school. This was not an easy decision for us to make, but we thought it would help his morale, so we allowed him to go. In a very short time it was necessary to readmit him back to the hospital. The illness continued to only worsen. No one seemed to be able to find the reason. Fear was a constant part of our lives in the weeks and months ahead, which lengthened gradually into years.

We were told that Edward should be taken to a hospital that had a children's ward and that more tests should be performed. We then moved him to another hospital that had such a ward. There Edward was transported by wheelchair down a long corridor, into an elevator, up several floors, and into a huge room. We couldn't believe our eyes, seeing so many children in a single area. They seemed so sick, so forlorn, all those lonely and unhappy children. We had thoroughly believed that we were doing what was best for our young Edward, but we knew that if we left him with all those sick and unhappy children, and with our limited visiting privileges, he would just give up. My husband, daughter, and I knew that this was no place for Edward, who looked so frightened. He seemed to shrink away from what he saw. He grasped my hand and spoke in a voice that was little more than a whisper: "Mom, do I have to stay here?" I felt as if I had lost my voice, but finally I was able to tell him that we were going home.

Even though our child was showing no sign of recovery, we took him home. Our worry and anguish were taking a dreadful toll on all of us. We tried to be hopeful, but we had little reason to foster that hope. When our desperately ill young son would try to smile and ask, "Am I doing all right?" we tried to be reassuring. It was difficult to do when the road ahead was becoming darker and darker. As we carried him to our car, I prayed and prayed that we were not making a terrible mistake.

My precious son! His condition was such that we began to fear that we had made a serious mistake in bringing him home from the hospital. At the suggestion of a friend, we made arrangements with a doctor, whom we did not know, to see Edward. This good man came directly to our home. After a limited examination, he said that Edward should be hospitalized and should have a thorough checkup. We were very fearful that Edward would not have the strength to endure another thorough checkup.

He then entered Edward into the hospital, where he stayed for five weeks, undergoing test after test and taking many different medicines. I spent almost all of my time with my child. I was in his room day and night, the five weeks he was there. Because he complained many times that his back hurt so badly, an X-ray examination was finally done. A diagnosis of compression fracture of the lower spine was made, and, after questioning by the doctors about any injuries he might have experienced during games, it was decided that the fracture might have happened when he had fallen while bowling, a long time earlier.

Medication after medication, in large doses, was given to Edward. In two weeks his condition worsened, and in five weeks he was no longer able to see or move himself from his bed. One day Edward barely whispered, "Mom, I came here with a backache, and I can tell my insides are very sick. Please get me out of here." I'll never forget a doctor at that hospital who called me out into the lobby and said, as if it were an ordinary statement, "Your son will not live to be sixteen. You should be glad you have had him this long." When I heard this, I felt weak and trembled and a hatred came over me for this doctor who lacked any compassion whatsoever.

Again we took our sick boy away from a hospital and returned home. We were leaving that hospital still with a very, very sick child and no diagnosis. He could not see, could hardly move, and was miserable with a rash of some kind all over his face and body. We took him out without a diagnosis or any suggestion that Edward be taken to some superior medical center for examination. We had no knowledge of any of the renowned medical centers, such as Johns Hopkins or the Mayo Clinic. At that time we believed that our local doctors and hospitals had all the knowledge that could be expected.

Maybe God's way of answering my prayers was to give me the strength to keep hoping that, despite all we had experienced, somewhere we would find someone who had the capability, the knowledge, and the experience to direct our child to recovery. We didn't know who, where, or how, but we continued to believe that we would find someone who really cared and who was capable of saving our son's life.

CHAPTER II

A Giant Step Forward

Our knowledge of renowned medical centers was not entirely lacking, but it was not sufficient to be of any use. What little we had was very limited and scattered knowledge, dreamlike, and not moving us to action. Our dear friends Mary and Sam Leto had told us about the Mayo Clinic in Rochester, Minnesota. Sam highly praised the clinic for the excellent care he'd received when he'd had his kidney problem several years before. They described the clinic as a wonderful association of doctors, comprised of groups of consultants in almost all fields of internal medicine, surgery, and research. The Letos urged us to take Edward there without delay. Why we did not respond to their suggestions more quickly, I simply do not know. After weeks of hospital experiences, frustrations, and growing fear, I guess I just considered the Mayo Clinic as a not quite real place.

It was Edward himself to whom the Mayo Clinic was real. Young as he was, he was amazingly aware of the seriousness of his illness and that his health was in no way improving. He really knew that he was almost hopelessly ill, and he had begun to believe that he would not survive unless there was a great change in the care he was receiving. From his hospital bed he said to me, "Mom, something terrible is happening to me. I feel worse and worse, and if you don't get me out of here, you will see my death notice in the paper. Please take me to the

Mayo Clinic. Don't listen to anyone. Just get me out of here. Remember what Mary and Sam said, that I'd have a better chance there to get well. Please, Mom, don't wait. I can't eat; I can hardly see; I hurt everywhere. Please, please, Mom, hurry and call the Mayo Clinic before it is too late."

My heart started to pound fast, and all I could think of was to hurry home and call the Mayo Clinic. I promised my son that I would go home and call immediately to make an appointment. I begged God to give me the strength and resolve to resist and overcome any obstacles I knew would be placed in my way. The general belief was that the physicians who had been involved in Edward's care had done everything that could be done to cure him. Some members of my family seemed to have accepted the feeling that he was not going to regain his health.

To this day I cannot understand why not one of the many physicians who had treated Edward had spoken to us even of the existence of a number of superior medical centers, including the Mayo Clinic. We learned about them later. I cannot believe it was lack of knowledge about such places. Perhaps it was ego that kept them from telling us.

"Your son will not live to be sixteen." The cruel statement that had been made to me by one of the physicians kept haunting me. In my prayers for a miracle I tried to rush home to make that call.

I went to the parking lot, found my car, and did not delay a moment in getting started. It seemed that every possible problem was placed in my way! In my great hurry, I drove over the cement divider that marked my parking space. What on earth to do now? I just got out of the car and ran as fast as I could the several blocks to my home. At my door I was horrified to find that I did not have my keys—that I had left them in the car.

I raced back to the car. My keys, fortunately, were there. I grabbed them and started running back home. I was in such a state of exhaustion and fear that I hardly knew why I was racing home. And I simply cannot recall how the matter of the car over the concrete block was resolved.

I became more and more worried, almost terrified, about making the call. I was sure it was the right thing to do to make the call and ask for an appointment. I was worried as to how Edward would stand the journey to Rochester. One question after another beset me.

I called the Mayo Clinic to explain to the best of my ability Edward's condition. It was such a relief when I heard the words that Edward would be examined as soon as he could be moved to Rochester. I was instructed to make the traveling plans and then make the plans known at the clinic so the necessary arrangements could be made to have an ambulance at the airport to take Edward directly to Worrall Hospital. Also, I would be given some assistance regarding quarters for me and those accompanying me.

To make matters even more complicated, we were experiencing an airline strike. Fortunately, my husband was able to make arrangements for a private plane that could accommodate our needs. As soon as there was a certainty about traveling, we took our son from the hospital, without the customary dismissal formalities from the administrative staff. They had made it very clear that we would be taking full responsibility for his care and that the hospital could not be held responsible for any flaw in his care.

Edward was so thrilled to learn he really would soon

be on his way to the Mayo Clinic that he truly believed he was going to be well again. Our hope was renewed.

The nurses who had taken care of our son were very nice and caring, but there was one who was truly outstanding. Her sweet smile, her loving sympathy, and her very gentle care of Edward gave us comfort. With tears in her eyes, she put her arms around me and said, "Mrs. Pompeian, we are all praying for Ed." We did sign a release form before leaving the hospital and heading home.

At home we had a hospital bed in our living room for Edward. I was terribly frightened to hear him say, "Mom, I can hardly see you." It filled me with despair. I wept as I sat at the side of his bed, hoping that he did not really know the depth of my fear and grief. Reaching to touch me, he found the tears on my cheek and tried to tell me that all would be well because we were going to the Mayo Clinic. Being totally exhausted and frightened, I got up to go across the room to sit in another chair to spare Edward my condition. My daughter came by me and said, "Mom, don't worry; I'll take care of you and Edward." All I remember was Sharon helping me to my room.

The decision to make the trip to Rochester after we got Edward's release from five weeks of hospital stay in Michigan and making the arrangements to admit him to the Mayo Clinic took a heavy toll on all of us. My whole family was very frightened, but they were glad that Edward was on his way to the clinic. My mother was always encouraging me, but now she remained silent. She told me later that she was very afraid that she would never see her dear grandson alive again. I grew more and more frightened, but I kept telling myself that he would regain his health.

Sharon was a great comfort and support for me and

for Edward. Over and over she urged me not to worry, adding that Edward would soon be getting better. She was sure he would be well again, and she told her brother and me that she would take care of us.

CHAPTER III
A New Adventure

It was April 1964, and we were going to take our fourteen-year-old son to the Mayo Clinic in Rochester. After we made this serious decision, there remained many things to do in preparation for our trip. How thankful we were for the caring and assistance of our dear neighbors and loving family members. Sharon was a marvel of help. She made it her special responsibility that everything was done to make us ready for the trip.

The night before leaving for Rochester, I put all of Edward's many medicines in a large bag to take with us. It was an incredible collection of medicines, each one to be administered on its own schedule. I kept a chart to be sure that I was giving Edward the right medicine at the right time. Also, there was the need to spray his throat after his every effort to swallow food.

The evening before we left for Rochester, I was exhausted. Edward seemed to be sleeping restfully, and I just had to sit down for a few minutes to get myself together to pray that God would watch over Edward and all of us. I wondered why we had to go through such a long painful and despairing time. As I sat and prayed, I felt a warm certainty that God was carrying us to a place where we would receive His special aid.

I twisted and turned and slept fitfully off and on that night. I would leave my bed frequently to check on Edward and then return to try again to sleep. Finally I fell into a deep sleep and dreamed an unforgettable dream—not a dream, I decided, but a vision. Our Lord appeared, holding out His hands to me. He said, "Take this." I could only see His hands reaching out to me and His white flowing robe. As my hands reached His, a ball of glowing light appeared in my hands and then slowly faded away. It seemed to leave me with new strength, strength that I needed badly to cope with all that happened later that same night.

The doorbell rang, and at first I thought it was a sound in another dream. But it rang and rang and finally I was awake enough to recognize the sound. I didn't want to open the door, as it was very late. I turned on the porch light, peeked out from the edge of the curtains, and saw a policeman standing there. I opened the door. My husband also was standing there. Facing this in my state of nervous fear was terribly difficult. I could only gasp, "What happened?" As they entered the house the officer explained that my husband had been in a car accident, but luckily, he was not injured. The car was totally demolished, but he was spared injury.

We did not go to bed for some time. There was so much to talk through about the accident and about the trip to Rochester, which now was only hours away. I checked on Edward and again found him sleeping quietly. There was little need to return to bed. I knew that I was too upset to sleep. I went to the kitchen and warmed a glass of milk. As I sat at the table sipping it, I reviewed all that had happened and all the unknown things ahead of us.

In due time we dressed for our journey to the Mayo Clinic, had our breakfast, and made ready for our farewells. The last evening we had packed everything we thought necessary to take with us. I had to tell my mother about my "vision." I had a peaceful feeling inside me. She said it was a special blessing, a promise of good fortune.

The ambulance came to take Edward to our chartered plane. He had to be flat on his back on a stretcher. Many neighbors gathered to wish us well, assure us of their love, and promise many prayers for the young boy whom they held in affectionate regard. It was with gratitude and a full heart that I said good-bye to my mother, others of my family, and friends.

At the airport Edward was lifted into the plane on one side where he would lie. Sharon sat near him, and I sat beside him to administer medication as I had been instructed.

An ambulance met us at the Rochester airport. Our pilot said good-bye to us and then said to me, "Take care of yourself." Edward, Sharon, and I were taken quickly to Worrall Hospital, where Edward was hurriedly taken to a room all ready and prepared for his arrival.

The condition in which they first saw Edward was a great shock to them. His whole body was covered by a reddish itching rash, his vision was intensely blurred, his speech was slurred, it was impossible for him to retain food, and he was unable to walk. I felt so sorry for my son, there aren't enough words to tell how his condition affected me. He was short for his age and suffered from obesity, skin changes, severe muscle weakness of arms and legs, and skeletal changes called osteoporosis. Their laboratory tests and kidney biopsy showed no evidence of lupus nephritis. The steroids appeared to be causing very severe complications and were discontinued.

After a short time the doctors felt that care for Edward's extremely serious condition could be administered in a better way at Saint Marys Hospital, also in Rochester. They took him off all medications, which the

Mayo doctors believed were actually making his condition worse. At Saint Marys Hospital he was treated with the greatest care and he began to show some hopeful signs of recovery.

After all the time Edward had been a patient in many hospitals in Michigan, finally a diagnosis was made—glomerulonephritis, an illness that has many forms. In Edward's case the form was advanced renal failure. One of his kidneys was totally nonfunctioning. The other kidney was functioning at only one-quarter of its strength.

One of the first and extremely important of treatments was the establishment of a very rigid diet, one from which Edward could not deviate for many years.

The arrival in Rochester, Edward's quick entry into Worrall Hospital, and then, a few days later, his transfer to Saint Marys Hospital seemed almost a dream to me. So much had happened in so short a time. I think I must have been numb both emotionally and physically.

I could not resolve the anger I felt toward the doctors who had cared for Edward through the many months, with test after test, surgery after surgery, and an unbelievable series of medicines in variety and quantity. All the time our son was becoming more and more frail. Never once did a single one of the many physicians who cared for him suggest that he should be taken to a major medical center. To our knowledge, not one made any effort to consult with any specialist in any field of medicine about the "mystery" of Edward's condition. The flat statement made by one doctor, "Your son will not live to be sixteen," was to me only an admission of their lack of ability to help him regain his health. That he survived their battery of tests and other endless treatments is a miracle.

My young daughter, Sharon, continued to give me the greatest kind of help. She was strong and loving, helping me through so many hard and terrifying hours, and once in Rochester, she understood that I still deeply needed support.

The Mayo doctors were very kind to me. They had many questions, of course, and I answered them to the best of my ability. Having Edward in their care gave us some peace. They told me, as I painfully knew, that he was extremely sick, but that they had every hope for his recovery; however, it would take a long time for him to regain even some of his strength.

After a few days, one of the doctors asked me if I had noticed any change in Edward. I told this doctor that I was sure I had seen some increased signs of alertness. He assured me that he, too, had noticed such signs and that it was very encouraging.

Even though I spent long hours at the hospital, I had a hard time sleeping at night. My thoughts were racing with reasons for hope and also with lingering fear. It helped me relax somewhat to look back at the kindness and love of my mother and all our relatives and friends who gave us loving comfort and assistance when we were preparing for the trip from home to the Mayo Clinic.

One of my dearest friends, a devout Catholic, gave me spiritual health, and she was lovingly kind to Edward. She prayed for him regularly and offered to give me holy water to use, as it might help him. I was very happy to have it.

My friend told me to touch Edward with it and add some to the liquids he drank. She taught me a prayer that she believed would be helpful to me and to Edward. Faithfully I sprinkled the holy water on the pillows and put a few drops in his water and milk or touched him or his surroundings with it.

I thought about telling Edward, and when I did tell him, he said, "Mom, I knew about it all the time." All that while I thought he didn't know what I was doing, and I was pleased when he told me and said he thought it was a lovely gift from my friend.

Each morning when I went to visit Edward, the nurses put him on a cart where he had to lie flat on his back. I would take him up and down the halls, and most of the time he wouldn't say anything. I had hoped that this action would liven his interest in his surroundings.

Then, one day, he said to me, "Mom, I am feeling a lot better, and everyone is so nice to me. Why don't you go home?" When he said that, I knew he was no longer frightened and he wanted me to get rest. He, as always, wanted the best for me and others.

My room was across the street from Saint Marys Hospital, a room my husband had found for me so that I could be close to the hospital. I was at ease a little, because I believed that Edward was out of danger and in the hands of the Mayo doctors.

CHAPTER IV
Progress and Worry

My whole pattern of life, from the beginning of my son's illness, was totally foreign to me. I had enjoyed a happy and more or less carefree existence with my family. I was young, unworldly, immature, and painfully unprepared for the abrupt change that serious illness brought to our family, physically, emotionally, and spiritually.

All the good things that were happening to Edward at Saint Marys Hospital should have been calming to me, but I just could not unwind. Of course, things happened that were upsetting. Mostly, however, the doctors and nurses were wonderfully good to him and to me. When the days came that I was allowed to take him, flat on his back on a cart, up and down the corridors, we were immensely pleased and encouraged. My fatigue, however, did not lessen.

I had been allowed, from the beginning of Edward's time at the hospital, to remain with him for many hours each day and on into the night. I knew I was not getting enough rest, but I knew, too, that it was best for both of us that I be with or near him as much as possible.

In preparation for the trips in the hall, the nurses placed Edward on a hospital cart, his means of transportation. I was always on hand to take him on his outing. His back was excruciatingly painful, and moving him onto the cart required very gentle care. One day as I was waiting, he screamed in pain in a way I had not heard before. I rushed into the room and said something like: "Be careful! You know he has a terribly painful back." The nurses looked at me, and one said, "We're trying so hard not to hurt him anymore."

The cart trips, up and down the hallways, had begun to spark Edward's interest. He saw other children in various stages of illness. Some were confined to their rooms, the activity of others was similar to his, and some were well enough to be in the playroom. Edward and I slowly became a little acquainted with some of the children and their mothers.

A happy thing had happened before Sharon had to leave me to return to school. One of her good friends, a really nice young man, paid us a surprise visit. He flew in from Pontiac, bringing Edward a gift he would keep into adulthood. It was a football bearing the signatures of all the players of the famous Detroit Lions team and a fine inscription to Edward, dated 1964.

I stayed with Edward until nearly ten o'clock that night. He knew I needed rest and kept urging me to go to my quarters and try to sleep.

I went downstairs and sat in the hospital lobby for some time trying to get a grip on myself. I tried to read but was just too tired to concentrate enough to have much of an idea about what I was reading. I simply needed to talk to someone close to me, so I called one of my sisters in Michigan. She was sympathetic and asked all the right questions about Edward, but she totally missed my need. I was upset and hurting, and she couldn't even sense how stressful my life continued to be. I put the receiver down without saying good-bye and went back to sit in the lobby. I was so dejected it frightened me. Just then I felt a gentle touch on my shoulder and someone said, "Mrs. Pompeian, are you all right?" I simply broke into sobbing, unable to answer. This lovely, caring person was one of Edward's nurses. She gave me great comfort as she listened to me. She talked with me long enough to help me get back in control. She knew how worried I was about my son, and she sympathized. She also knew that my need for rest was beginning to be serious. She reminded me of the progress Edward was making and that the doctors were encouraged by the progress. She told me she would be his nurse the next day and that I should try to relax enough to really manage a night's sleep.

I hope this wonderful nurse understood how grateful both Edward and I were for her very special kindness. When she left me, I went out to my room. I crossed the street, paying absolutely no attention to the cars that were passing by. I thought of stopping at a restaurant across from Saint Marys but I had not remembered that closing time for these places in this area was early, so I went on to my room. A group of women were visiting in the living room. They invited me to join them, but I thanked them and went on to my room for another sleepless night. Very good news came to me in the morning. My sister May called to tell me that very soon she would be joining me for a number of days. She gave me even more good news: our mother would be coming later to spend time with me.

CHAPTER V
Better Times

It's a wonderful feeling to greet a new day as a day of promise—a promise of better times ahead.

It was a beautiful morning. As I went to the hospital, I felt certain that something good would happen. I entered Edward's room to see a light that I had longed to see was shining in his eyes, and I knew he could hardly wait to tell me something really exciting.

"Mom," he began. "Mom, I know I can sit in a wheelchair! I'm going to ask my nurse if I can. I know she will think it's a good idea. And then will you take me down the hall so I can play pool? I want to play pool with some of my new friends!"

The promise I had felt in the early morning was being fulfilled! I finally knew a feeling of gladness. I had almost given up hope that I would ever hear such a statement or such a request from Edward. The nurses were also pleased, and the wheelchair was allowed on a trial basis. The new venture was wonderful therapy in morale building. He became an eager and cheerful visitor. As I wheeled him through the hallways he had fun telling me where to go, and he thoroughly enjoyed exchanging greetings with those we met in our travels.

The playroom was very well furnished to provide safe and entertaining activities for children of all ages. As a meeting place it was truly special for the youngsters. They made new friends and found many ways to have a good time, as good a time as their health would allow.

Edward and I visited other children who still were bound to their rooms. Edward's dormant sense of humor was coming alive, and he found he could make them laugh or, at least, smile. This, of course, pleased him and delighted me.

Near his room a little Korean girl was confined to her quarters. She was only five years old. Her illness was leukemia. She was a tiny, fragile child, with beautiful huge dark eyes and shiny dark hair and a lovely smile. We visited with her and her parents frequently, and Edward always enjoyed seeing her laugh or giggle at his jokes and quips. He was so sorry that she was so sick. Sometimes she would beg her parents to take her to his room so she could laugh and have a good time.

One morning when I was helping Edward get ready for our travels through the halls, he solemnly asked me to do something for him. He was worried about his little friend as she became more and more fragile. He wanted to give her a present, something he hoped she would like. He thought she would like a doll. We talked about it and decided that a doll was a present she would really like. I went shopping, and he liked my choice. He asked one of the nurses if he could go to the little girl's room to give her the pretty cuddly doll. The nurse was sure that his visit and his gift would make the girl happy. So we went to her room and found her awake.

Edward couldn't wait to give her the doll and, almost at once, sang out his cheery announcement: "I brought you something! Can you guess what it is?"

She smiled and said, "Something nice! Can I have it, Eddie?" She was delighted. She held out her little arms to receive it, then held it close and hugged and patted it.

Her parents and Edward and I watched her happily. She kept saying, "Look what Eddie brought me! Look what Eddie brought me!" It was a heartfelt moment as all of us saw her pleasure. At the same time we could see how her strength was waning. Edward and I were happy that his gift had brightened her life for even a short time. Her pleasure was shared by her parents, who knew what little time remained for their precious child. This short visit gave Edward and me much to consider about his illness and how wonderfully his health was improving. Together we said a prayer for his little friend and a prayer that our blessings would continue.

The days and weeks went by. The doctors were pleased with Edward's progress. He was gradually gaining strength, and they began to speak of a possible time for us to go home—maybe in a few more weeks. They could not predict at all about when he might be able to walk. We all knew that happy time was a long way away. Our days were spent in a fairly routine hospital pattern.

Edward was seen and tested by many doctors. After he had been in the hospital for some time, therapy designed for strengthening weakened muscles was begun. This included walking between bars where he gradually learned to support himself, always with a therapist at his side. This became a vital part of his daily treatment.

We continued our wheelchair trips in the corridors, taking longer routes. We visited other children and their parents, and, of course, we frequently went to the playroom. He enjoyed playing pool, which he was able to do in an awkward manner from his wheelchair.

I thought many times of our family and friends in Michigan, but strangely, I was never homesick. I was lonely, sometimes desperately lonely, but I felt that my home was with my child.

Finally, after eight weeks, we left Saint Marys Hospital to return to our home in Pontiac. We agreed with the doctors that we would return to the clinic for follow-up examinations as they thought necessary. I thought as we were traveling, of the incredible difference between Edward's condition at this time and his terrifying condition as we traveled to Rochester two months earlier. I knew God had heard our prayers, and over and over again, I sent my heartfelt thanks to Him.

After a brief rest following the journey, and after being so joyously received and greeted by our family and friends, it was time to begin another phase of working toward recovery.

CHAPTER VI
Life Back Home

It took some time just to get settled back in our home after being away from it for so long.

Many decisions had to be made about how our time would have to be scheduled to accommodate Edward's general, but crucial, care and therapy. It was his good fortune that he no longer had to take any prescribed medicine. The medicine now was his strict diet. The preparation of this diet was more time-consuming than one would expect. It meant shopping so all the right ingredients would always be on hand, as well as arranging for the planning and cooking time.

Naturally, everything about Edward's treatment had been decided by the doctors at Saint Marys Hospital over the long time he had been a patient there. A back brace had been designed for him because of a compression fracture. It was considered likely, because of the kind of injury, that it would be necessary for him to wear the brace for approximately six months. Once home, we had to follow these decisions. Careful and gentle care was required in removing and replacing the brace, because of both the pain and his very sensitive skin. This particular care was only one part of the overall care.

We had been home only a few days when a terrible tragedy occurred, one that totally overwhelmed Edward with grief. He and Eddie McKerricher were playmates, schoolmates, and dear friends for most of their lives.

They had made plans for the future to travel together to many places when they were out of school. Planning to see Eddie again as soon as possible when we were home was foremost in Edward's thoughts. When we received the shocking news that Eddie had drowned, Edward was heartbroken. I was fearful about how dangerously this deep sorrow might affect his recovery. He absolutely insisted that he be taken to the funeral home and to the funeral. I couldn't let him know how opposed I was to the further trauma or why such an undertaking could be very damaging to his physical and emotional condition. He said he wanted Eddie to have something from him. Edward asked Sharon to take him to a jewelry store to help him buy a small gold cross for Eddie to wear.

We finally decided that we would honor Edward's request to attend the funeral. We were fearful that either his going to see his friend or his being denied his great desire could be hurtful. So we went to say good-bye, and the cross was placed on Eddie. It took many days for Edward to recover enough from this shock and sadness to carry on with any energy.

Sharon attended the funeral with us. Friends and relatives of the devastated family from many communities were there for the services and at the home after the burial. There was, of course, a general mixing of the guests. In the tradition of the Armenian culture, dinner was served.

On this occasion Sharon met a young man with his grandparents from Detroit, Michigan. This meeting was the beginning of the romance that led to their marriage.

It took a long time for Edward to recover from his grief enough to want to even think of his many games, collections, and toys. One day he told me that he had no further desire to keep them. Some things he chose to give to friends. Otherwise, he chose to sell all but a very few that he really wanted to keep for himself. Then he decided to have a sale. He wanted an ad placed in the paper. He developed a unique system for selling. Everything for sale was placed unpriced in our recreation room. Once a choice was made, the buyer would go to Edward's room, where he then would decide the price. Obviously, his prices were accepted as totally fair, because some of the buyers returned for possible further purchases only to find all items had been sold.

In due time we had to consider Edward's stepping back into some kind of school arrangement. We worked out a plan that was more or less satisfactory. There were consultations with the teachers he had had before the onset of his illness. They came to our home to renew our acquaintance and evaluate Edward's alertness and interest. It was easy for them to see that he was eager to get involved with classes. The decision for the early resumption of his schoolwork was simple but effective. A tutor came to our home to work with Edward on assignments made by his teachers. The tutor stayed with him for a designated time and then left the work with Edward for his review. I then returned the assignments to the teachers for their evaluation. We followed this routine until Edward became physically strong enough to attend school.

The sessions of therapy were not adequately satisfactory at one of the hospitals. It was necessary to resume his program of recovery at another hospital. These periods of therapy had to be held for some considerable time before we could even think about his actual return to school. An attendant from the hospital would come and pick Edward up from his bed and carry him to the van, and when therapy was done this attendant would bring Edward and me home.

Edward and his father had a game they played when Edward was beginning to take a few more steps by himself. After his prolonged illness, his dad promised him that as soon as he could walk more strongly into the living room, he would earn a new color television set.

This was a very good stimulus. Edward worked at taking more steps but was very careful not to overdo. It was not long before he earned the television set in color that he had so anticipated. It was a very happy addition to his life.

There was a joyous happening the week before Christmas. The music teacher, for whom the youngsters had great regard, brought Edward's class to our home to sing all the lovely Christmas carols. Edward was very surprised and enjoyed their coming, so delighted they had done this for him. It brought back memories of his singing in the choir. We, of course, invited the whole group in for hot spiced apple juice and festive cookies.

It was a wonderfully happy day when Edward was taken back to Washington Junior High School, which was so full of memories for him. He soon began to feel that he really belonged in school, and he did very well in working toward making up the work he had missed for such a long time.

The time went by very quickly, and all of a sudden it was graduation time from junior high school. We knew, of course, that Edward would be unable to be in the procession of graduates approaching the stage where the diplomas would be presented to the students. It pained us that he had to be deprived of this pleasure. It was very nice that the school's principal delivered the diploma to Edward at home.

Then it was on to high school. The first problem at Pontiac Central High School was the need to use the staircase, with its many steep steps. We realized very soon that Edward could not manage too many steps, up or down. We made the necessary arrangements for his attending another school that eliminated the problem of steps.

So we moved Edward to Pontiac Northern Senior High School, where he was able to move about without the obstruction of steps. It didn't take very long for him to find his way about comfortably and begin to become acquainted with his new classmates and teachers.

Through all the years of Edward's illness, even when he was desperately sick and almost without hope of recovery, he did not lose his love for learning and his belief that someday he would be well enough to return to school again.

High school was a whole new world filled with unfamiliar classes, new requirements, and students that were beyond the young-boy status. Edward learned very quickly that adolescence was a new stage in his life, and he liked the feeling of growing up. His health was such that he was physically unable to do many things the other students could do. The schedules of therapy and rest had to be observed, but they did not deter him from his class preparation, which he did diligently. These school years passed pleasantly, considering his delicate health. He did not deviate in any way from his early style of study.

We received a letter dated May 13, 1969, from Mr. Philip J. Wargelin, principal of Edward's school, that brought us great joy and pride in our son's accomplishments. The letter stated:

It is our pleasure to advise you that your son, Edward, has been elected to membership in the National Honor Society at Pontiac Northern High School. This selection was recently made by a faculty committee on the basis of demonstrated qualities of character, service, scholarship, and leadership. Kindly accept our congratulations on this significant achievement, for this is a credit to you and the home which is represented. . . .

CHAPTER VII

A Whole New World

A wonderful thing had happened to us. We were all deeply thankful, happy, and proud, and Edward was thrilled and excited. He had graduated from high school with honors! From the early days of his illness we had been given little reason to believe that we actually would experience this kind of joy.

Here he was, a young man eager to step into a whole new world of higher education and much more that he had never been able to know. He knew, of course, that there were many health problems always to be considered, but he had developed a true talent for convincing himself and the family that he would do very well away from home. He promised that he would always be near a telephone for emergency use and that he would be very careful of his limitations.

Edward's first venture into the new world began in the autumn of 1969 at Adrian College in Michigan. He was very pleased to know that on the campus there was a chapel where he could go and pray.

He found life in a dormitory where he lived to be lively and fun. All went well with him until the spring of 1970, when he became ill again. He was knowledgeable about all of his health problems and knew that this illness would take him back to a hospital, so he called home.

I had never heard him sound so dispirited. I told him I would leave immediately. I remember his saying, "Mom, you know your sense of direction to get somewhere isn't all that good. Please be careful." I told him that I would watch all the signs and that he should not worry. I hung up the phone and went out to the car. I looked in my purse to make sure I had some money in case I needed it. I only had a few dollars, so I ran back into the house, grabbed my checkbook, and ran back to the car, thinking all the time, *Hurry. Get to Adrian as soon as you can.* I started the car and only could think, *I have to get to him fast.*

I am a very careful driver and obey traffic rules, but as I kept thinking that I must hurry because of what had happened to Edward, I pushed harder on the accelerator and drove like mad. I kept hoping the police would not be looking for me. Then, after several hours, I began to wonder why it was taking me so long to get to Adrian. I stopped in Jackson, Michigan, at a gas station and asked the attendant where I was in relation to Adrian. I got all flustered and nervous when he told me that I was many miles away from Adrian and I had to backtrack. I couldn't believe what I had done.

Trying to hurry to get there, I had missed Adrian, and now Edward would be so worried about me and wondering what had happened, knowing I should have been there much earlier. At the station I told the attendant to please fill the gas tank.

I had begun to see that I was in serious need of gas. He filled up the gas tank. I signed the check, asked him for detailed instructions to Adrian, and really drove off faster than before. I was vaguely aware that he was quite amused. He probably was thinking, *There goes another stupid woman driver!* All I could think of was: *Hurry and get to Adrian.* I truly don't know how, but I made it.

Edward had been very worried. The first thing he said to me was: "Mom, did you get lost?"

I just said, "Are you kidding? I sure did. I went all the way to Jackson, Michigan, where the state prison is."

I don't know what else went on in his mind, but I was very glad to be able to take him home. All of his things were packed. His friends put all of his belongings into the car and bid him good-bye, and we were on our way home.

When we got home my husband asked me, "Did you write a check?"

I said, "Of course. I was almost out of gas."

He told me then that a call had come to our home asking for a Helen Pompeian who had written a check in the checkbook of someone else by the name of Sharon. How I got her checkbook and where my checkbook was at that time are beyond me. My husband told me that he had told the caller that another check would be sent to him. All I know is that I had to get my son home. That was my only thought.

My first thoughts for Edward at home were to make him comfortable and urge him to rest. I decided to call one of his doctors at the Mayo Clinic and describe what had happened and that it was necessary to bring Edward home. The doctor's conclusion was that all of the new experiences that had made up Edward's college life had been overly stressful and that extreme fatigue was the result. He urged several days of complete rest and told me that if there were no improvements in Edward's condition, I should call him again. We followed this advice and we lived relatively comfortably through the summer.

In September 1970, we believed he was well enough to begin his second venture into college life at Oakland Community College in Farmington, Michigan. He chose this college because the doctors suggested keeping him close to home. He chose courses that would take him into law and business administration. He was named "Superior Student" there and was able to enjoy his classes, his classmates, his professors, and reasonably good health. Then came the next terrible blow!

In the spring of 1971, Edward suffered a seizure and collapsed. He was rushed from the college to a hospital close to our home. We are forever grateful to the caring people at the college for sending Edward directly to a hospital and informing us immediately.

We had a talk with one of the doctors to say we felt that Edward should be transferred to Ford Hospital in Detroit, Michigan. The doctor was worried and said, "Go ahead, but I think you are making a mistake by taking him anywhere right now. He is a very sick boy." I told my husband and family why I thought we should take Edward to Ford Hospital. It was important to me because I knew one of the doctors there.

I called Ford Hospital and told them of Edward's condition. They made arrangements for his transfer. Our ailing son was on a merry-go-round of hospitals. At Ford Hospital he was examined and the decision was made to put Edward on peritoneal dialysis. Our young son never complained to us, but I am sure down deep he was a frightened young man.

I stayed with my son at Ford Hospital night and day by his bedside until arrangements could be made for my husband and me to learn how to run the dialysis machine when Edward was released from the hospital.

This was the most frightening treatment that Edward had received through the seemingly endless time of his illness. Yet this treatment was necessary to save his life. This was in the early days, when there was little availability of kidney machines.

No anesthetic was given while they did the peritoneal dialysis. A dialysate solution was alternately being infused into Edward's abdominal cavity, then removed to cleanse the impurities from his blood. That night he said to me, "Mom, I am so cold." He kept turning his head from side to side and told me, "I can't stop my head from moving." Right away I went down the hall to the nurses' station and told one of the nurses. She said she would send someone right to Edward's room.

It may have been minutes, but I thought it was hours. No one came and Edward's condition was worsening. So I went again, and this time growing more upset, I told the nurse to get someone immediately, that he was so cold and he couldn't stop his head from moving side to side. Finally a nurse came and then a doctor shortly thereafter. They found the dialysate solution going into Edward was not working properly and he was receiving cold instead of warm solution and that the Compazine medication was causing his involuntary head movement. Compazine had been given to him earlier because he was sick to his stomach.

He was frightened and told me, "Mom, please call the Letos. I want to see Sam as soon as possible." I found a phone and began my effort to get in touch with Sam and Mary Leto. Unfortunately, I did not have their unlisted telephone number with me. I told the telephone operator about the urgency of the situation and that Sam Leto would want to know about the serious condition of his "fourth son." She was unmoved and even refused to place a call to them herself to ask them to call me, so I returned to Edward's room.

In a shorter time than one could believe, I looked up to see the Letos in the doorway of the room. Edward exclaimed, "Oh, Sam!" After I recovered from the incredible surprise, I asked my dear friends how they had happened to come to Ford Hospital. Had the telephone operator softened enough to put in the request? Sam simply said that he and Mary had had a strong feeling that Edward needed them. They called my home—no answer. They called three different hospitals—no knowledge of Edward. Finally, they found us at Ford.

Their coming was wonderfully good for Edward. The visit of these devoted and caring friends lifted his spirits immeasurably. They made daily hospital visits for almost a week, until the doctors at Ford Hospital made arrangements for Edward to be seen in the kidney unit at another hospital, the only available unit, also the closest to our home, that had a limited number of kidney machines. My mother and my two brothers were with me at the hospital and were always there and of great support to me. Sharon and my sister Janet came faithfully to be with Edward and me all the time we were there.

CHAPTER VIII
Slow Progress

On our arrival at the hospital we were directed to the small lobby of the kidney unit. We were surprised and startled to see many patients sitting there, some looking worried. We wondered, of course, why they were there. We eventually learned that an evaluation was to be made on each of those present, an effort to make careful estimations of who of the patients could receive the greatest benefit from use of a kidney machine.

God blessed us. Edward was one of the patients selected. His treatments were initiated using the Travenol artificial kidney machine. The treatment was commonly known as dialysis. It was administered six hours a day, three times a week. The Scribner-Quinton shunt was used for access to his circulation. Three times a week we traveled the thirty miles from our home in Birmingham to the hospital, where the treatments were continued for three months.

Because of the very high cost of the hospital treatment and because we knew that it was necessary that the treatments be continued for a long time, not yet determined, we knew we had to make plans for having the treatments at home. During the three months of Edward's treatment, he and his father learned all the fine details for use of the Travenol. Some considerable changes had to be made at home for installation of the

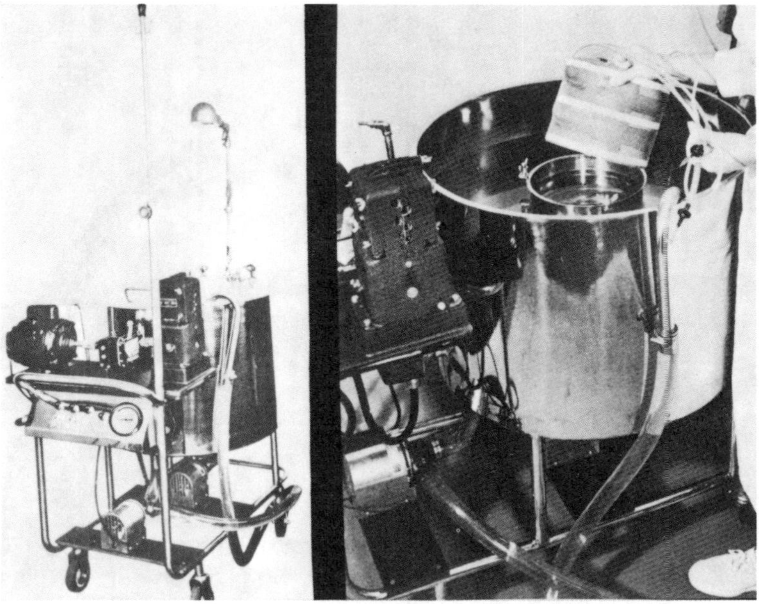

Type of artificial kidney machine used in North America from 1960 to 1970. This kind of machine was used in Edward's treatment.

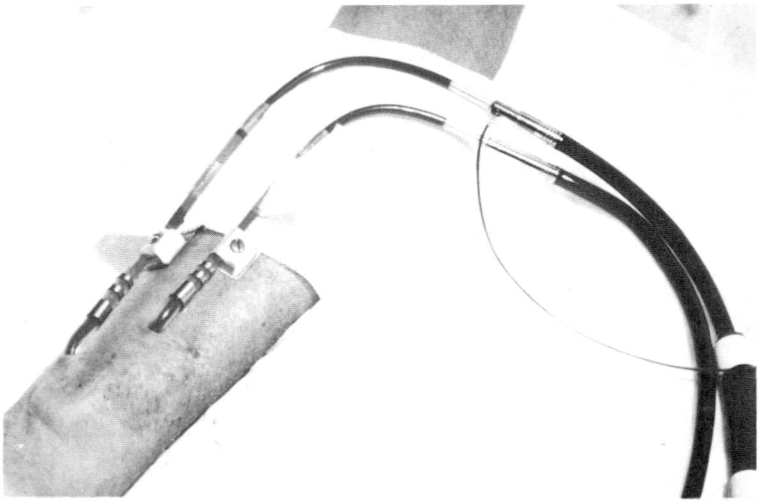

Type of external access to the circulation used from 1960 to 1970. Heparin was given during treatment. Between treatments the plastic tubes from the artery and the vein were connected by a plastic shunt to prevent clotting of the blood.

machine. Treatment at home would be on the same schedule as at the hospital.

My part in this home system was to prepare the equipment for use. This involved taking care of the dialysate solution and being very careful that its temperature was correct. After each treatment I did thorough cleaning and sterilizing of all parts of the machine, which was extremely important.

My husband had learned very well the method of handling the treatment. A shunt that was permanently implanted in Edward's arm accommodated the two tubes that circulated the blood through the machine, after which the system cleansed out the impurities that his almost nonfunctioning kidneys were unable to remove. The treatment at home required constant supervision to prevent life-threatening accidents. Use of the equipment or the shunt practiced at that time has been discontinued for a long time. Edward and I would go to the hospital once a month to pick up supplies.

It is hard to describe the incredible misfortunes that were part of the use of the shunt at the hospital. It is enough to say that many scars and much scar tissue on Edward's arms from the efforts made to insert the shunts will never disappear. One of the incisions was most painful. He suffered such pain and near torture during these insertions that I still shiver when I think about it. I still don't understand how my son tolerated the incisions that were made, but he always was able to endure the pain. Serious infections also were results of the handling of the shunts, and hospitalizations were often required.

During the two years of treatment at home we learned a great deal about the love and goodness of so many people—members of our family, friends from the earliest days of Edward's illness, and new folks who had just become friends. So much help and support was offered. Even members of the Birmingham police and fire departments made themselves acquainted with our home, where Edward spent most of his time. In case of fire or any violence, they planned the best way to care for him.

Despite my worry about Edward's health, I really became rested, rested to the point of being able to accept the invitation of the National Kidney Foundation to be chairperson of a committee to organize and carry on a fund drive for the foundation. I knew so well that much research was in progress, but that much more was needed in the further recognition and treatment of the dread life-threatening kidney disease. Halloween candy attractively packaged to sell for one dollar a bag was sent to us by the foundation.

My neighbors, my family, and the great number of Birmingham residents who participated were simply wonderful—people of all ages, including children from the very young into adolescence—and amazingly, we all had fun selling the candy. When the big truck delivering the candy rolled into our driveway, it was an exciting event. The fund-raising went on full-force until every one of the innumerable bags of candy was sold. We were thrilled and proud of our accomplishment when we learned that our drive was one of the top ten in Michigan, and this was Birmingham's first involvement in this type of drive.

Obviously, Edward was unable to do any door-to-door selling, but he wanted to participate in all the excitement. He became our treasurer and did a masterful job of handling all the money.

At the end of two years of dialysis at home, we decided that it was time for Edward to be taken again to the Mayo Clinic.

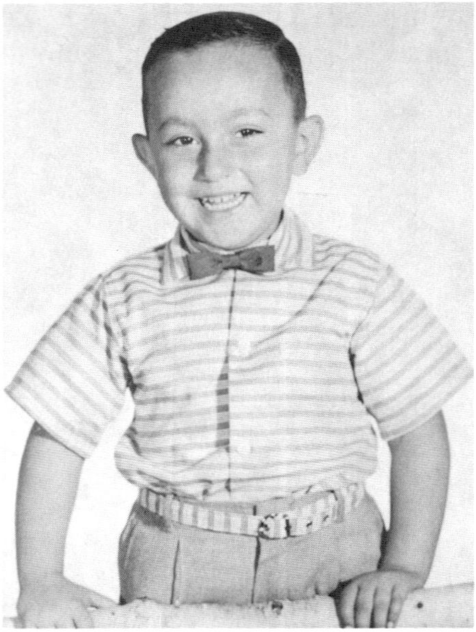

Edward, a happy, healthy child.

Edward at graduation despite the severe and lingering illness.

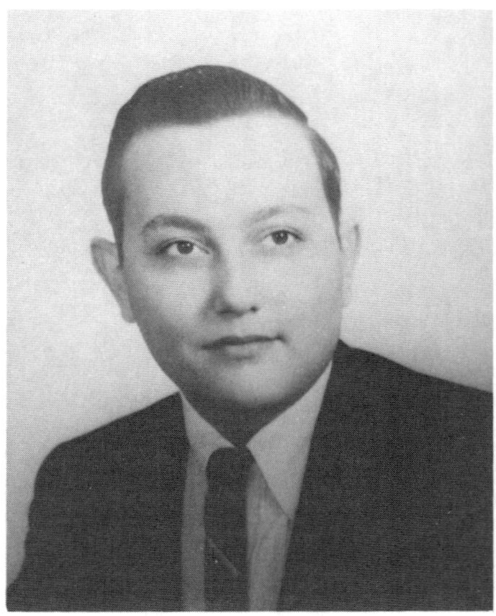

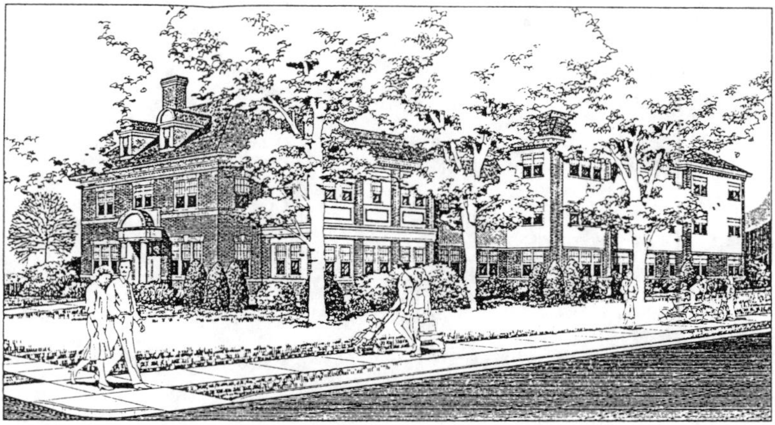

New Gift of Life Transplant House, as drawn by architect Christopher W. Colby, AIA of Yaggy Colby Associates.

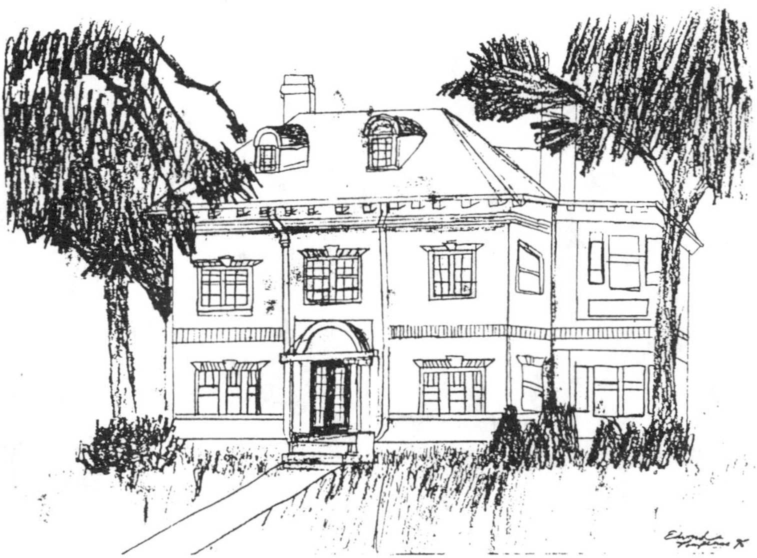

Gift of Life Transplant House, drawn by my eleven-year-old grandson, Edward. Obviously he has a fondness for trees.

CHAPTER IX

Exciting and Fearful Times

The first dialysis at the Mayo Clinic and the examinations by the doctors clearly indicated that a very long stay in Rochester would be necessary. Again the same schedule for dialysis was established, six hours a day, three times a week. Time and treatment were needed to prepare Edward for removal of both kidneys, which had become totally nonfunctioning. All of us, especially Edward, were very relieved and in much better spirits now that he was in the care of the Mayo doctors.

We began a search for a home that would be reasonably comfortable for Edward, Sharon, her son, little Paul, and me, and fairly close to the clinic.

Edward missed his friends in Birmingham greatly. He had been well enough to go out with them occasionally to favorite restaurants where they could enjoy talking, planning for other outings, and good food. They even had double dates once in a while and would go to an amusement park or a ball game, have a picnic, or see a movie.

While Edward was dialyzing he could concentrate on class preparation and read any number of a variety of stories, articles, and books. Best of all, he could enjoy visits of friends there with him or by phone.

Sharon assumed the responsibility of finding a place where we could live. In two weeks she found a nice apartment that would satisfy our needs very well.

A number of patients and Edward were being dialyzed at the clinic at the same time. They were all in the same area and were placed close enough to one another to allow them to begin to become acquainted. Edward rallied his sense of humor, and before long he really was amusing them.

Edward would tell jokes or relate some of his own funny experiences. And, with his encouragement, he soon had the other patients telling their own favorite stories. Just in fun, he presented the idea of having lunch brought in once in a while for a change from routine food. It seemed a great idea to all of them, but they could see problems. How could such an arrangement be handled? Edward quickly assured them there would be no problem. He'd write notes about each one's desire, and his mother would be glad to take care of the whole situation. I couldn't refuse, as I wanted to do anything I could for my son and his friends. It gave me a good feeling to be able to do this for them and to see that they made a real party of this deviation in their routine.

I think of those many friends often when I remember Edward's condition after dialysis. He would be weak and sometimes light-headed. Little Paul was always eager to help with pushing the wheelchair when it was needed. Also, there were fierce muscle spasms sometimes in Edward's legs at unexpected times.

Sharon will never know how much her love and support meant to me and Edward. She understood, of course, that we were deeply grateful, but such feelings are not easy to convey. This time in Rochester was a very unhappy and difficult time for her. She was experiencing the sad days of divorce proceedings. It was an extremely stressful time for all of us. The marriage that had had such a promise of happy and mutual devotion had collapsed, with little hope of reconciliation. Sharon and I were both greatly worried about Edward, and she, of course, was worried about me and worried about her own situation. It is possible, I believe, that all she did for Edward and me gave her some helpful distraction from own problems. She was like his guardian angel.

The total change in our lives, living in a new and strange city and separated from the many members of our family and our wide circle of friends, was hard on all of us. I found myself back in a state of constant fatigue and disturbed sleep. I had begun to have strange and upsetting dreams that seemed to have no possible connection to our current lives.

Of all things, I dreamed about the Armenian massacres. I had little knowledge of those horrors. What I knew was mostly from our family history. Horrible tortures and death of thousands of Armenians were perpetrated through many years of Turkish brutality. My parents, totally unknown to each other at that time, by some miraculous means escaped these atrocities, although many of their relatives did not. My mother, only sixteen years of age, and her Armenian friends who lived in a home that Mother's parents owned somehow managed, in terror, to move through Constantinople, now named Istanbul, and find their way to a ship to travel to the United States. We are not certain about how my father escaped. When he arrived at Ellis Island, there obviously were no objections to his entering the United States. He entered this country with plans to join his sister in Pontiac, Michigan. My mother, of course, also arrived at Ellis Island. Relatives met her and took her to Pontiac. She met my father, Nicholas Nazarian, shortly after her arrival. At that time the Armenian population there was limited, and any new Armenian people arriving were quickly made welcome. Some were married within a short time.

In my dream I suffered all the agony of the massacres and lived through it as my parents did. This dream recurred a number of times, and I always awakened from it in overwhelming fright. I almost hated to try to sleep for fear that the dream would happen again.

Time is so strange. Sometimes the days and nights fly by, and other times they seem endless, unkind, depressing. We were in these days approaching three very serious surgical procedures, and we experienced many varieties of the caprices of time.

Edward's illness and Sharon's wretched problems were always foremost in my mind. Taking care of the home, preparing the food for Edward's strict diet and a different menu for the rest of us, watching the times for the trips to and from the clinic, watching over little Paul when his mother, now a registered nurse at Saint Marys Hospital, had to be away from him, and many other needs—laundry, shopping, incoming and outgoing mail—kept me so busy, so tired, and so worried that I feared I would become totally worn out. My sleep patterns were not providing the rest I so badly needed. Even so, we managed a fairly reasonable life.

Rochester, Minnesota, home of the world renowned Mayo Clinic, is an extraordinary city. It offered many diversions that were of interest and help to us in increasing our sympathy for and empathy with others.

As time passed we learned more and more about the clinic and the city. We were truly fascinated. People came from all over the world to bring their health problems to the famous medical center. In the clinic and hospitals and the city's places of business and streets we saw many ethnic groups; many styles of clothing; people in conspicuous bandages, casts, and braces; people walking with canes, crutches, or walkers; and those being transported in wheelchairs. And we heard many languages.

The transient population was large. There were, of course, many hotels, motels, restaurants, and stores to accommodate these people and their companions. And there were Saint Marys Hospital, Methodist Hospital, and Olmsted County Hospital.

The doctors were pleased with Edward's progress. They knew, however, that he faced a number of surgical procedures through September and October. The operations were as follows: September 15, nephrectomy, appendectomy, and removal of spleen; September 19, bronchoscopy; September 26, abdominal exploration; October 1, gastroscopy; October 22, limited abdominal exploration and drainage of peritoneal fluid.* How he had the strength to survive all that he had for so many years is a total mystery to me. I really do believe that miracles, together with all the wonderful professional care he finally received, gave him the willpower and strength to live.

The legal matters of Sharon's divorce were finally concluded, and it was so good for all of us to be relieved from that strain.

My weariness, however, continued, and I could not free myself from constant worry. My sleep disturbances continued. Dreams always nagged me—strange dreams full of action, sad dreams with tears, and then the nightmares. I longed for a quiet, gentle night's sleep.

*Dr. John E. Woods and Dr. Franklin J. Leary performed much of the original surgery, including the transplantation from me to my son.

Time passed more quickly than we expected, and suddenly it was time to make plans for Thanksgiving. Edward, with Sharon, little Paul, and me, made great plans together. Dialysis friends who were here without family were warmly invited, of course. The festive day came and I proudly served a bountiful and traditional Thanksgiving dinner. We and our guests felt especially blessed to be able to spend this time together. They enjoyed the number of hours in pleasant sociability and made certain I knew how glad they were to be with us and how greatly they appreciated the delicious food.

CHAPTER X

More Exciting and Fearful Times

Edward, Sharon, and I had been very reluctant to tell our family and friends in Birmingham, especially before holiday time, of our earlier major decision to reside permanently in Rochester. Christmas always was a beautiful and special day for us. We finally decided that we would announce our plans on New Year's Day so we could celebrate that day together, a day that gave us not only hope, but total belief that God would make 1973 the greatest year we had known since 1963. The operation for Edward's kidney transplant would be accomplished, and we would be forging into a new and wonderful life for Edward and for all of us. This we truly believed.

We knew that when our decision was known there would be an emotional response, with tears and remonstrances and, finally, loving prayers and good wishes. Our news, coming on the first day of the year that had such promise for us, eventually became more acceptable and reasonable to all our family and friends.

Shortly after New Year's Day it was time for us to return to the Mayo Clinic for further preparations for the transplant. The first necessary step was to resume the dialysis schedule, six hours a day, three times a week.

For some time we had felt the need for a different apartment, one that would give us the space we wanted for more comfort and, we hoped, a little privacy. Sharon, of course, undertook the responsibility for finding a better place for us. In a very short time she was successful.

Moving always is a pesky job, regardless of how simple it might be. It took several days to prepare for the new apartment, and our moving there was a fairly easy event, with no complications. We wanted to be well settled before a date for the transplant was decided.

A happy surprise came to Edward shortly after we were moved and settled. A couple of his schoolmates had some free time from college and decided to visit their old friend. They traveled from Michigan to Rochester by bus during a very, very subzero time. It was so cold that the bus could offer no real comfort. When they finally arrived at our home, they were so cold that they wondered if Rochester was located at the North Pole. The joyful reunion and endless quantities of good hot food soon had them pleasantly comfortable. Their visit was brief, but it was wonderful medicine for Edward.

Some serious complications followed the surgical procedures Edward had had in the fall of 1972. At the time of the removal of both kidneys (nephrectomy), his spleen and appendix also were removed. The later problems were pneumonia, pancreatitis, and delayed wound healing, all of which delayed establishing a date for the transplant. However, we were filled with hope and prayers that the time for the transplant could be settled before a long time had passed.

Early in 1973 Edward had begun to make real progress in gaining strength and recovery from all the setbacks.

From the time that we first learned that he was being considered for a transplant, my constant and greatest wish was that I could be his donor. His doctors knew how much I wanted this—anything to help my son. Many tests were arranged for me, some of them completely unknown to me. To be accepted as a donor, total physical compatibility with the patient is absolutely necessary.

We had received only casual information that a date for the transplant really was being considered. One day after the dialysis, young Paul was wheeling his uncle down the hall, ready to make the easy trip home. Sharon and I were following close by. It was midwinter and so cold that we were especially glad the distance was not great. Dr. William J. Johnson and Dr. Richard D. Wagoner, two of Edward's very special doctors, were coming in our direction and stopped us with what I expected to be a small exchange of a few pleasantries. After a brief conversation, Dr. Johnson asked, "Have you heard the good news, Mrs. Pompeian?" I told him we hadn't heard anything special. Then he said, "We have scheduled April 26 for Edward's transplant." This was stunning news that we had hoped to receive for days and weeks and months.

Sharon also had indicated to Dr. Johnson that she hoped to be Edward's donor. He told us that if I passed all the tests, I would be the donor. About donors he made a statement that we won't forget: "We'll take the best donor. This is not a competitive matter."

It's hard for me to describe my reaction to this long-awaited news. I was thankful and relieved. I was panic-stricken and could not hold back the tears. Our years and years of prayers were leading us to this great day. God's goodness and mercy had brought my son through dreadful years of illness to this time. We were certain that this date was a promise that great good would come to Edward. How could we think otherwise?

After working through all the emotions, I finally remembered that April 26 was Paul's birthday. I thought then when Paul was older he could think that for this birthday he had received a most wonderful gift, the day of the beginning of his dear uncle's new life. Of course there would be some celebration of Paul's birthday on a day when all of us could enjoy being together.

Since the date, April 26, had been chosen, I knew it would not be a long time before my tests began. If I were not an acceptable donor, it would be necessary to test others. I do believe in my heart my prayers were answered.

I was totally unprepared for the need for a psychiatric examination for both my son and me. When I learned the reasons for it, it was not too hard to understand. To begin, it is imperative that a donor does not have a deep fear of the surgery and that the offer to be a donor is made because of a true desire to give the patient a chance for better health, maybe even for life. The donor must desire to do everything possible because of compassion for the patient. Was pressure placed on one by the family or friends to do the *right* thing? Was the offer made because of a feeling of guilt for some earlier hurtful action? I had dreaded a psychiatric examination, but I passed through it satisfactorily.

My only reason was my love for my son.

Then when terrifying dreams began again to give me miserable and restless nights, I knew I had to learn some way to calm myself. The old nightmare about the Armenian massacres did not recur, thank heaven. It was replaced, however, by a dream about a horrible and heartbreaking accident that had devastated my mother and her young family. It happened when I was just a little girl, eight years old. It was about my loving and gentle father, who was killed in a terrible train accident. In the dream I was no longer a child but an almost grown-up teenager. I was at the scene of the tragedy, seeing the gruesome results of the accident and feeling that it must be my fault. I was alone, terrified, and filled with grief—alone with not a soul there to comfort me. The dream haunted me a number of times, and I tried and tried to understand this horror coming into my life after all the years from childhood to grandmotherhood. It never was possible for me to settle on any possible reason for the revival of my upsetting and sad thoughts about my father. I remembered what my mother had said about my father, that he was a very caring and loving person and one for whom his family came first.

I often wished my father could be with me to comfort me. I believe I told Sharon of my wishes. Such wishes might have been the base of the dreams.

CHAPTER XI
The Crucial Date

There is no doubt but that members of our family undertook to be on hand to encourage and support Edward and me. Having had their loving care and concern through so many years, we knew many of them would be with us before, during, or after the surgery, at times we most needed them. And, of course, Sharon was there and my brother Paul, my sister May and her husband, my sister Janet, my niece Diane, Alice Tashjian and her sons, and Armine Jibilian and her brother, Ardag. My mother, brother Richard, and sisters Alice and Isabelle kept in touch by phone as well as close friends and relatives.

One night, shortly before the time of the transplant, I had a most wonderful dream. I call it a vision—another vision—and to this day I truly believe that I had the exquisite experience of a vision. Edward and I were sleeping in the same room. Our Lord walked between our beds, and His flowing robe touched us softly from head to our toes as He lifted His arms, blessing us. I moved quickly to Edward's bedside to awaken him. I told him about my beautiful dream. I told him that this lovely visit was a message to us that everything would be all right. Edward, barely awake, said, "I hope so, Mom."

The day before the transplant, I was scheduled for the final one of the big tests. This had to mean that the results of the other tests were satisfactory. I was sure that this test was expected to be satisfactory, too. I was hospitalized overnight for the arteriogram dye test. The dye was injected into the aorta. The test gave an indication of the function of the kidneys and the entire arterial anatomy of both kidneys. This test was to determine the state of both kidneys, that both were functioning normally, and that I could live well with one kidney.

So came the day of the transplant. I was wheeled into the operating room. Edward already was there in another operating room. I felt no fear of the surgery that would be performed in the next few minutes. Edward and I had absolute confidence in our surgeons. Dr. John E. Woods and Dr. Franklin J. Leary were primary transplant surgeons.

I awakened in a strange room, hearing someone calling my name. It took some time to collect my thoughts, enough to think then: *Transplant*, then: *Edward*, then: *What are we waiting for? When is the operation going to begin?* I must have asked the questions aloud, because someone told me the astounding news: the operations were completed, and both Edward and I had gone wonderfully through the whole process. We were in recovery rooms, where we would be monitored carefully for some hours.

I hadn't been awake long when Sharon, all excited, came into my room to tell me the great news: Edward had begun to void ten minutes after the graft of the new kidney was completed. We joyously thanked God for showering us with His choicest blessings.

Fortunately, the graft functioned successfully, and I experienced no complications. It never ceases to amaze me that somehow we had struggled through all those necessary years that finally brought us to this time.

The postoperative recovery for both of us was remarkably uneventful. Some of it for Edward seemed almost impossible. He was allowed to eat solid food after surgery, on the same day! He was allowed to sit up and was encouraged to walk on the same day! It's hard to believe that that is the way it was. After the transplant he was in the hospital for three weeks, and he left feeling wonderfully good and delighted to be free from the dialysis of three years. It was necessary for him to have three checkups a week for some time.

Dr. Woods was extremely pleased that not only did Edward do very well immediately following transplantation, with no serious problems in the immediate post-transplant period, but went on to become an extremely independent, productive, and very successful human being, both as an individual and in business as well. In his case, the renal transplant seemed to signal not just a return to good health but a complete turnaround from the standpoint of his independence and functioning. In April 1974, about a year after his transplant, he underwent a secondary procedure to drain off an accumulation of fluid, and he recovered from this uneventfully. From a medical standpoint, he continued to do very well from his renal transplant in the years that followed.

One of Edward's favorite pronouncements was: "So far in my life since my illness began, everything that is good has happened to me in Rochester."

Because of the effect of steroids, which he continues to receive in small doses to prevent rejection in addition to the high doses he received during puberty, he has continued to have skeletal complications. He is short in stature, sixty-one inches. He still has evidence of osteoporosis, and has suffered a number of fractures. Efforts to improve his calcium metabolism have included removal of several parathyroid glands and subsequent treatment with vitamin D. Despite his many problems, he continues to be active physically and in business and community affairs. Through all of this he never lost his good humor and his gratitude for his gift of life.

Our time in Rochester was very lonely and stressful for me and for Sharon and Edward. After years of loneliness and experiencing my husband's indifference, I decided that a legal separation would be best.

CHAPTER XII
A Whole New Life

By the time Edward was released from the hospital and during those weeks when it was necessary that he return to the clinic three times a week for examination, we were well into spring. I don't remember that springtime had ever been so wonderful since the springs we enjoyed when all of us were well and happy, before 1963. Edward had more than survived the transplant surgery. He had never been so happy, and so it was for me. My most heartfelt prayers had been answered. My son had lived and it was my joy to have been his donor. One time he said to me, "Mom, you have given me life twice!" All of the beauties of spring were magnified for us—bluest skies, loveliest weather, exquisite flowers, and all. We were blessed.

Edward began to find himself thinking and talking about college and thinking about enjoying some kind of interesting work sometime in the not-too-far-away future. As spring and summer progressed he spent many hours with old and new friends who were awaiting their transplant experience. He frequently invited them to our home for visits and sometimes for lunch or dinner. No elaborate meals were planned. It was just the sociability that was important. They talked, laughed, and exchanged their health reports. They mostly enjoyed being free from the clinic or hospital environment for brief periods.

Beginning in the fall of 1973 Edward resumed his

time in college. He attended both Saint Teresa's College in Winona (he was the only male student) and Rochester Community College, where he attended science classes that would be helpful in preparation for his part-time work in the microbiology laboratories at the Mayo Clinic. This was to be his first real job.

During his attendance at Saint Teresa's, he had an efficiency apartment and drove back and forth to Rochester weekends for his work in the labs. After a time he became ill and was very disappointed that he was unable to return to his classes or to the microbiology laboratories.

It took more time than was expected to readjust his medications to support his stabilization.

After looking for work for some time and finding the search unsatisfactory, Edward decided he might like real estate. Eventually he did join a realty firm in Rochester and was sure he had made the right decision.

Shortly after Edward had begun his work, he called me to say, "The broker of the firm is in need of a secretary, and I told him that you are an experienced secretary. He is waiting right here to talk with you." The sum and substance of the whole matter is that the broker asked me if I was interested in the job. I decided that I was interested, and he asked me to begin the work in their office at my earliest convenience, adding that there was no need for an interview.

Edward was not long in the business before he acquired a following of his own clients. One of the clients, Daryl Engelhardt, became very important in Edward's life.

In due time we decided that we should start a search for our permanent home, and it was Edward who found it. He was so pleased that he couldn't wait to have me see it. He, Sharon, and I experienced love at first sight, and little Paul did a thorough job of exploring.

We decided that this really was our home. We were so fortunate that the house was in beautiful condition and we were able to occupy it as soon as such a move was possible.

We hadn't lived in our new home a very long time when misfortune struck us. Edward was preparing for work one morning when his hip gave out on the staircase and he fell the whole distance. He suffered acute pain and was unable to move or allow anyone to help him move. I called the ambulance immediately, and he was taken directly to the Saint Marys emergency room. I was in no condition to drive, and a friend came to take me to the hospital. When I found my way to Edward's room, I was so relieved and happy to find Daryl there at his bedside. I thank God that no broken bones resulted from the accident, which probably had happened because of the weakness of his left hip joint. It was so good that the disablement did not last for a long time. He rested at home as long as he felt it was necessary.

It was during this time that Edward developed the idea of establishing his own practice, with its headquarters at home. The house was so designed that his office needs could easily occupy space at the lower level and not interfere with the privacy of the home.

CHAPTER XIII
Work and Travel

We had become well experienced in adjusting to every change in our lives, and there had been so many. Here we were, Edward and I, becoming acquainted with the intricacies of real estate. Neither of us had had any idea at all about the complexities of the business.

To do the job the way it should be done, one must want to do it and have knowledge, diligence, patience, skill at handling public relations, and willingness to work any and all hours—all of this among other capabilities. Also, one must be licensed after passing state examinations. Edward was accepted in the firm as a valuable member.

His visits to the patients waiting for or having had transplant surgery continued. Those visits were a dedicated part of his life. The friendships that developed were deep and steadfast. One family, Luis and Angela Uribe from Colombia, South America, made frequent trips to Rochester and the clinic during the long time that Luis was being treated to be prepared for transplant surgery. Luis and his wife, Angela, and Edward spent lots of time together, and the Uribes became frequent visitors in our home, among the many others who came. There always was fun talk about when Edward would visit them in their country. We were always sorry when they left Rochester and always glad when we knew they were returning.

All went along very well in the realty business, and

Edward had a great thrill when he made his first sale, which earned him a nice commission. Earning differently from the hourly wage he had known before was quite an exciting experience.

A year had passed when I learned that a son of one of my dearest friends in Michigan had been killed in an automobile accident. I felt that I had to be with the parents in Pontiac at this sad time. I was so grateful to my employer for giving me a generous leave from the office. Of course, I spent several days with my own family, but I was unable to enjoy any relaxation and I could not rid myself of feeling apprehension. I called Sharon in Rochester several times to ask how she and little Paul and Edward were getting along without me. She assured me that all was well with each of them. Something in her voice or her manner of speech made me certain that all was not well. I made arrangements to return to Rochester at the earliest possible time and called Sharon to give her my flight schedule, knowing, of course, that someone would meet me.

Edward and a close friend, Chuck Parker, were at the airport when I arrived. When I saw Edward, I just about crumbled with fright. He looked so pale and fragile, and his right arm was in a miserable cast. My first thought was that the bandages were supporting a shunt in his arm and that he had lost his kidney. I burst into tears and could not stop my sobbing. Chuck put his arms around me, trying to calm and comfort me. Then I blurted out the question: "Did he lose his kidney?!" Edward told me about the accident while Chuck went to get my luggage, and he said, "Mom, I am OK. I really am fine!"

A bad car accident had happened right in a business section of downtown. Edward had entered the intersection on a green light when a driver in a heavy car ignored the red light and came crashing through into Edward's car, totally wrecking it. That he and his companion escaped death was a miracle. Edward suffered cuts and bruises, and his arm was very badly injured. When I learned the whole story I was deeply surprised that the injuries were not far more serious. Some time passed before he was able to return to work, and then, of course, there were many limitations on what he was able to do because of the broken bones in his right arm. It was more than necessary that he continue to use his cane to maintain his balance.

In the fall of 1976, Luis and Angela returned to Rochester for Luis to go through his routine of examinations. This time they were more insistent than ever that Edward pay them a visit. They wanted him to spend the January of 1977 with them in their city, Medellín, Colombia. After much eager planning, it was decided that Edward would begin his trip to join them on December 29, 1976. January is not the most robust time of the year in real estate.

Flying from Rochester to Miami and then on to Medellín was pleasant and uneventful. Happy time really began when Edward stepped from the plane in that city.

CHAPTER XIV
Special Learning

Edward's loving friends Angela and Luis Uribe and a nephew and his wife were on hand to greet the Uribes' American friend. It was a wonderful and joyous reception. As soon as the luggage was extricated from the many kinds of traveling gear that had arrived, Luis guided Edward to customs and made short work of moving him through with no complications. Obviously Luis was known and had influence.

Driving to the Uribes' home was really exciting. Everything was completely different from anything Edward ever had witnessed. He had been told much about the city of Medellín, its people, places of business, cars and other means of transportation, and the beauty of the countryside. All that he had been told had not prepared him for what he saw in those first few hours of his visit.

A fabulous party had been planned, and very soon after arrival at the elegant home, the party was in full swing. Many relatives and friends were there. Massive bouquets of exquisite flowers were everywhere, and the food was unbelievable to see and to taste. After Edward's quiet lifestyle, it was incredible that he was to experience all of this in one day until the end of the party. It was like a dream of a fantasy world.

The guests were saying good night to one another, and for those remaining, retirement time was welcome.

Edward rested very well and was not disturbed. When he was ready for a new day he joined the family.

Angela and Luis had every day of the whole month of Edward's visit planned. He marveled at such arrangements. Very early in the visit Edward was treated to a most extraordinary event. He had known the Uribes for a long time and knew very well that Luis had a great sense of humor and could produce unbelievable situations at most unlikely times. They were highly regarded guests at a special occasion in the small city of Guarne. The mayor and city council of that city were honoring the mayor of Medellín and her staff, of which Luis was a member. At the meeting impressive introductions were made and there were many speeches. When the time came for Luis, he, of course, spoke his thanks for the warm greetings and fine reception. Then he introduced Edward as mayor of Rochester, Minnesota, USA. As a mayor, Edward was given the royal treatment. The speakers in their messages especially addressed Edward, and one gave him a brief speech on the historical background of Colombia's fight for independence. No one questioned that the very young man could hold such a position. Luis thoroughly enjoyed his caper and the attention given his guest and proceeded to translate what was said about Edward from Spanish to English. Edward was shocked and surprised. "Leave it up to Luis," he said.

Among the festivities that were part of the day, the Queen of the Day for Guarne was crowned. Luis had arranged for her to travel in his car to a favorite restaurant chosen for further formalities. Edward was seated beside her and enjoyed her smiles to him and to the people along the way as she waved her hand to them.

Back in Medellín they had a party for the police force. Everyone had a great day. The many people who were attending were loving every minute of the music, dancing, and drinking. The people in Colombia Edward found to be very hospitable and very happy.

The next few days were celebrations for the New Year, and Luis and Angela, with their family and Edward, visited the home of Luis's brother Raoul and his family and then they joined Angela's family. All were warm and friendly and hospitable people and obviously had great affection for one another. The parties, the food and drink, the music and dancing went on and on with never a sign of fatigue. Edward marveled at being a brief part of what seemed to be pure joyousness.

Edward was shown about the city, Luis's businesses, and the mountains and thought this must be one of the most beautiful places in the world. Edward clearly saw the social division in the population. The people were either very wealthy or very, very poor, and they lived accordingly. There was no discernible middle class. He wondered if the wealthy felt much concern about those families living in their sad squalor. He saw people on the streets who were ill and disabled, and he thought about his friends in Rochester awaiting their transplant organs. He thought how wonderful it would be if each of them could have a donor soon and recover from the transplant surgery without complications. He thought of the whole new world that could be waiting for them.

Edward was diligent about keeping his diary up-to-date. There were so many lovely people entertaining him in so many ways that it was necessary to write daily résumés of the activities. They spent time shopping in fine stores, eating in the best restaurants, going to beautiful churches and museums, and there were always parties in the planning. He had hours of just seeing and feeling all the aspects of life in Medellín as Luis and Angela knew it.

The most dramatic event of the whole visit happened during the visit to Bogotá. The cable car ascent to the top of Sarate Mountain, 11,000 feet in height, was spectacular. There at the top was a beautiful shrine, famous for recoveries from illnesses and disabilities for visitors who were suffering.

The day of the visit was beautiful beyond words. Edward felt himself part of the blue sky, the sunshine, and the feathery clouds, and he experienced a profound sense of spirituality that he never lost. Many had left their canes, crutches, and wheelchairs at the shrine. After prayers Edward felt a wonderful feeling of peace and relaxation. Six months after his return home, he felt no need for using his cane.

The descent of their cable car, from the mountaintop back into the city, was the beginning of the end of his wonderful vacation. They took time to witness a bullfight and joined in all the excitement that was everywhere. Edward was truly sad that he had only a short time until the time of farewells.

The return to Medellín gave him only a few hours to finish his packing and take off for the airport. After embraces with those who had accompanied him, he was in the plane and taking off for Miami and home to Rochester.

Angela and Luis continued their frequent trips to Rochester and the clinic for the tests and examinations that were regularly scheduled for Luis. Much of their free time they spent with us, and our friendship deepened with each visit. They persisted in their invitation to me and my family to visit them in Medellín as Edward had. A date finally was decided: August 22, 1978. Edward,

Sharon, little Paul, and I were all excited and pleased about what we considered an exotic adventure—this wonderful trip to Medellín, Colombia.

A fearful thing happened that made us wonder if we could or should go on this trip. We experienced a real disaster for our city, its surroundings, and many, many people during the night of July 6, 1978. With little or no warning, nature can do terrible things to a community that had no warning or way of being prepared. There was a horrible rainfall, the heaviest in seventy-seven years, which flooded the city. A power loss caused a complete blackout and made radio and TV useless. The devastation to many homes and other properties left complete chaos. Our governor and mayor, viewing the damage, declared it the worst known in this area. Four people trapped in an elevator in a nursing home drowned. The elevator had descended into the flooded basement and could not be raised. The Salvation Army and Red Cross supplied their wonderful assistance for the homeless and injured. When we left to begin our trip to Colombia, so short a time after the massive damage left by the storm, we almost felt guilty to be going away for a good and happy time.

The journey from Florida to Colombia was, far from our expectations, anything but pleasant. During the long flight it was necessary to land, for what reason we didn't know, and where we were we didn't know. We were told only that it would be some time before taking off for Colombia. An hour later we were told there were mechanical problems and that it was necessary that we leave the plane. Still later we were told that we would be staying overnight. Here we were, bag and baggage, in a strange place and not knowing the language. Then we were trundled off to a hotel in another area where we would remain until the repairs were made to enable continuance of the journey. The bus trip back to the plane was beyond description. People and luggage were stacked in together, and the driver knew nothing of speed limits, going through red lights, or, we thought, of driving. It was clear that his only mission was to make the fastest possible trip to wherever we were going. Little Paul was the only one who considered the happenings hilarious fun. Arrival in Medellín seemed a marvelous accomplishment.

Angela and Luis and their family were there with their happy greetings to welcome us. Luis made little of gathering our luggage and moving quickly through customs. That he was a man of influence we could not doubt. We were whisked through the city to their lovely home, where we were treated like royalty by the warm welcoming party. The beautiful flowers and the enticing and bountiful buffet were only part of all that had been planned for us.

Plans had already been made for every day of our visit. The day after our arrival we went up into the mountains, where we were to meet and have lunch with Angela's family—a memorable day. We traveled in two cars, Sharon and I with Angela, and Edward and little Paul with Luis.

Both our friends clearly were skilled and fearless drivers. They zoomed up the narrow roads with hairpin curves that had no guardrails at incredible speed. I tried not to show that I was absolutely terrified. We asked about the wooden crosses that were posted along the roadsides. Angela told us that each cross marked a place where death had occurred because of an accident. In the little villages along the way Edward, Sharon, and I were saddened by all the evidence of dire poverty that we saw, and we wondered if any measures were being considered to help these people.

When we arrived at the meeting place, Angela's family greeted us warmly. What gracious people they were! We were taken for a walk around the small parklike area and were deeply thrilled looking out and at and over the mountains. I still remember my amazement to see such spectacular beauty.

We were served at a picnic table and suffered some embarrassment for not knowing anything about most of the food. There was such a variety. We enjoyed some of it and found some of it almost impossible to eat. Luis assured us that it took some time to acquire a taste for such unfamiliar food and that we were not to feel uncomfortable about not enjoying all of it. We had several hours of pure pleasure, and then it was time to leave these delightful people and return to Medellín.

Following Angela's plans, we spent time for a few days shopping and seeing much that made the city. Of course, there was a great party at a club to which Luis belonged. The sumptuous buffet offered food and drink hard to describe, and the hall was filled with laughter, singing, and dancing. It was exciting when the mariachi band came to our table to serenade us. At some point in the music we heard: "Sharon." Luis looked at her and said, "It's for you, lovely lady." One could not believe such a party without actually being part of it.

After some time, Edward told me he wanted to leave. I couldn't understand this. He had given no reason. I should have known that something was wrong. Angela took him home. It was the beginning of a frightening illness, and we knew that it was important to take him immediately to the Mayo Clinic, where his vast illnesses were completely recorded. We were sorry to leave our friends, but we knew it was best for Edward, for all of us, and for Angela and Luis that we leave for Rochester at the earliest possible time. I telephoned the clinic, and arrangements were made for Edward to be taken directly to Saint Marys Hospital. We thanked God that we made the right decision to come home. Edward was confined in the hospital for several weeks.

During this time, as he became stronger, he thought a lot about his future, about many things, how his business would grow, how his transplant friends were doing, and how good it would be to plan some social events.

CHAPTER XV
Relationships

We hear and read about meetings day after day, but it's a rare time that we give the matter much thought. Meetings and organizations are for reasons that are established—secret, business, happenstance, ridiculous, inconsequential, support, religion, politics, government, and hundreds more. And, of course, there are the groups who assemble for social times, reunions.

Soon after Edward had felt strong enough to begin some social organizing, he talked with a number of his transplant friends about one of his ideas—an annual reunion dinner. The idea was accepted with enthusiasm, and many entered into the plan.

Since follow-up tests and examinations were necessary once a year at the clinic, all agreed to plan their registration times early enough to allow them to meet in Rochester at more or less the same time each year, which included the time for the reunion. The date chosen was the first Sunday after Easter. This was the beginning of a wonderful relationship that lasted ten years. I was very happy to be included.

Groups of this kind usually include a few whose joyous and careless actions keep the party lively and entertained. One such delightful person was Gloria. Her favorite expression was, "Oh, well." Remembering Gloria was remembering, "Oh, well!"

On one occasion I agreed to go to the Minneapolis

airport to meet our close and very dear friends Dr. Artin Jibilian (who also was one of Edward's doctors) and his wife and children, who were returning to Rochester. It was going to be a tight race to make the trip and return to Rochester in time for the early mixing and exchange of greetings and the dinner.

Dear Gloria was full of enthusiasm, not only accompanying me, but to drive her car. As I have mentioned, my sense of direction is not very good. I told Gloria we were taking the wrong route. She was on the way to the Rochester airport. When I said we should be on our way to Minneapolis, she laughed and said, "Oh, well," and made a U-turn to correct our direction.

All of a sudden I noticed that we were approaching a red light, and Gloria drove right through.

I said, "Gloria, you just went through a red light!"

She remarked, "I did? Oh, well."

The traffic had increased as we drove closer to the cities and the Mendota Bridge, a huge bridge over the Mississippi River. We almost drove straight into the siding of an approach to the bridge. I didn't say a word. I couldn't. I just thought, *What next?* As we moved into the traffic, I didn't want to hurt Gloria's feelings, but I finally got enough nerve to tell her that she had to be more careful. She looked at me questioningly and said, "Oh, well."

When we found a parking space at the airport, I was relieved and thankful. Before going into the terminal, I thought it would be helpful to have the matter of the drive home settled. I said, "Gloria, I hope this will not hurt your feelings, but I must ask you something. Are you having problems with your eyesight?" Then she told me that her vision was not the best and that she was scheduled for cataract surgery in a week. My heart flipped over.

One thing after another happened. Our passengers could not be found. The paging system was loud and clear but brought no response. Then I tried telephoning, and I learned that our friends Dr. Jibilian and his wife and children had already arrived in Rochester and because we were late and their children were very tired, they had decided there must have been a misunderstanding, so they left to return to Rochester.

Gloria and I agreed that I would drive back to Rochester. Driving a strange car was hardly comforting, but we did arrive safely in Rochester in time for dinner and fun. Sharon and Edward were very concerned about our late return and wanted to know what had happened. I have laughed many times about that trip, and I made strong resolutions to have full knowledge of the capabilities and attitudes of any future traveling companion.

As always, the get-together was a happy time for everyone. Dinner was excellent, and for a considerable time later much talking and exchanging stories of the past year was thoroughly enjoyed by many.

CHAPTER XVI
Work for Kidney Research

For the first time in many years we were enjoying a truly calm period in our lives. I had begun to feel that I really wanted to do something in support of the Kidney Foundation in its research. Organizing some fund-raising events seemed the best way. Remembering the big monetary success and the fun of our candy-selling effort for this cause in Michigan in the earliest days of Edward's illness, I decided to try to organize a similar kind of action. I knew, from firsthand experience, the importance of the research, and I had some sense of how costly it had to be.

It took a considerable bit of time before any action could begin, but it did. Several groups of women in nearby small towns, especially Byron, were wonderful in their effort, and they collected a surprising amount of money. Then there was a group who canvassed in several of our shopping malls very successfully, as well as those who participated in door-to-door action in Rochester. The Kidney Foundation was very grateful.

Everything had gone so well that I began to have dreams of a far greater crusade. I received no encouragement to try so vast an action. I recognized that I had allowed myself to be carried away by our home successes. However, I still believed that better and bigger efforts could be made. Maybe someone widely known or famous, a celebrity, would accept an invitation to chair a fund-raising event in the Upper Midwest. I talked about it with many people who listened but offered no help or encouragement.

My sister Janet's in-laws, Helen and Edward Mardigian of Bloomfield Hills, Michigan, were the first to make me feel that such an action was one to pursue. They suggested that I extend an invitation to Mike Connors, star of the television show *Mannix*, a dear friend of theirs, giving him a brief summary of the purpose of my effort and my many years of knowledge about the work of the Kidney Foundation.

This was an exciting venture. As I wrote my letter to Mike Connors, I couldn't believe I was writing it. I thought there really was little likelihood of his accepting such an invitation, but I felt compelled to write it. I knew that he was well known for his work for charitable causes. I had heard that he was a very kind and caring person. I hoped that when he received my letter his response would be favorable. I briefly enclosed an account of Edward's illness and his kidney transplant, stating that I had been fortunate enough to have been his donor. In not too long a time, Mr. Connors's response did come to me. My son, daughter, and I were filled with joy that he had accepted the invitation.

I was amazed and terrified by all that had to be planned and accomplished—dates, locations, assistants, special guests, events, publicity, and endless other needs, including accommodations.

So came the day of Mike Connors's arrival: March 25, 1977. A small select group had gathered at the Minneapolis airport to greet and welcome our guest. All I could say was: "Mike!" when he stepped from the plane. I couldn't utter another sound for a few seconds. From the airport the National Kidney Foundation chairman, a few others, and I took him by limousine to his hotel. Later that evening, Mike, my husband, and I accompanied him to an elegant reception at the home of Dr. and Mrs. John Najarian. A Najarian son came to the hotel to take us to his parents' home.

Dr. Najarian was chief transplant surgeon at the University of Minnesota hospitals. He and his wife had planned this event for two heartfelt reasons. They had high regard for the Kidney Foundation of the Upper Midwest and they had high regard for Mike Connors and his Armenian heritage. His Armenian name is Krekor Ohanian. The guest list included sixty-five or so Armenian families from the area who were delighted to meet and greet our guest, a compatriot, a favorite TV star, "Mannix." Since we were with Mike, we also received a very warm and hearty welcome from Dr. Najarian and his family. Among those greeting us were Sharon and Edward, my sister May, and her daughter and son, who came all the way from Michigan. Dr. and Mrs. Arthur Bulbulian and Mr. and Mrs. Harry Tashjian attended from Rochester.

A feast of gourmet food was served. A lavish Armenian buffet, and beautiful music was provided by two famous violinists: Arsham Ohanessian and Henry Gregorian. And, too, there was Armenian dancing. At 11:00 P.M. Mike, my husband, and I said our good nights and left the happy party of Armenian togetherness.

Dr. Najarian presided at the testimonial dinner on Saturday, March 26, at the Marquette Inn in Minneapolis, where he introduced Mr. Connors as honorary chairman of the drive for the Kidney Foundation of the Upper Midwest. I thoroughly enjoyed being seated at the right of Mike at the table. Among the other honored guests were Drs. William Johnson and Iqbal Krishan from the

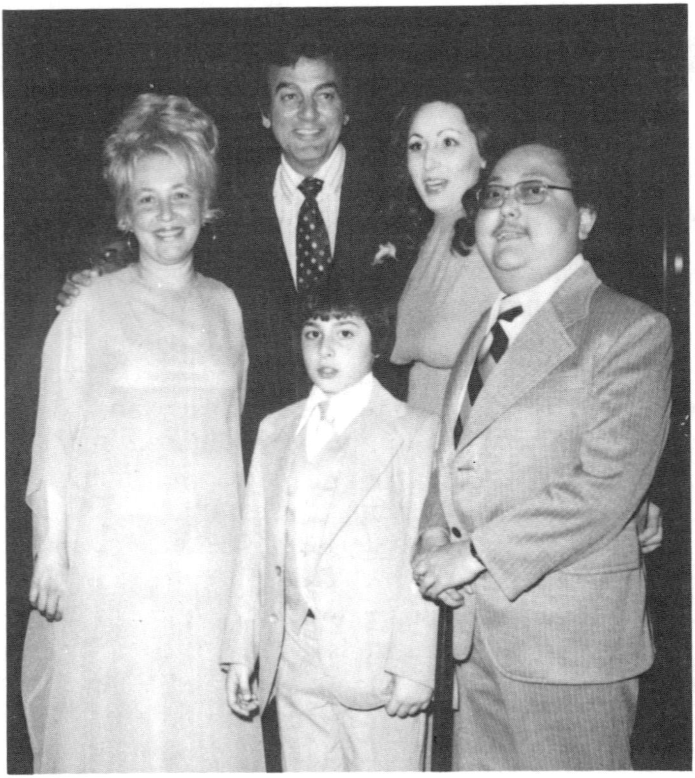

Mike Connors at I.D.S. Crystal Court in Minneapolis with me, little Paul, Sharon, and Edward.

Mayo Clinic and their wives. Edward, Sharon, my sister May and her daughter and son, Sandy and Bob Sexton, Daryl and his wife, Rita, and many people from Rochester were there together with people from the cities and surrounding areas.

Mr. Connors spoke, telling how deeply touched he was by the problem of kidney disease and how greatly he was impressed by the many dedicated people he had met.

A very warm letter with a generous donation was sent to me from Edward and Helen Mardigian, who expressed their regret to me and to Mike that they were unable to be with us.

After dinner there was a huge reception at the I.D.S. Crystal Court in Minneapolis, where an enormous crowd was being entertained and, more importantly, to greet "Mannix."

I was deeply impressed to learn of Mike's heartfelt interest in Armenian history and his acute knowledge of the Armenian massacres. His grandfather had been a victim of those terrible days.

Some time after Mike's generous visit to Minnesota, my family and I with friends were in California, where we attended one of the early presentations of Mike's movie narration, *The Forgotten Genocide*. He spoke of the inhumanity and the horror of the torture that killed far more than a million Aremenian people—men, women, and children. He spoke of his grandfather and what he had learned about his death. He ended his talk with the stern admonition that schools should be compelled to teach the lessons of man's inhumanity to man.

The genocides, Armenian, Jewish, Cambodian, and others, should be known in an effort to curb such horrible atrocities that even now could be in a state of planning.

CHAPTER XVII
Dream Come True

After Edward's recovery from the surprise and miserable illness that so abruptly ended the visit with dear friends in Medellín, Colombia, he put his mind seriously to the future. He realized that there could be health interruptions to any plan that he might consider, but he reminded himself that no one has a lease on life, even for the very next moment.

It was during this time that he concentrated on plans for establishing his own business in real estate, with headquarters at home. The house was so designed that his office needs could easily occupy space in the lower level and not interfere with the privacy of the home.

Obviously, he and Daryl had discussed this idea many times, and the more they thought about it, the better it seemed. They almost automatically became partners and eventually established Pompeian Englehardt Realty.

In the same year they purchased the Regency West Apartments, and business was off to a good start.

Through the time, before and after, Edward received his kidney transplant, he kept in touch with patients who were going through the traumatic waiting period to receive an organ, their hospital stay, and recovery. He visited them, encouraged them, and did everything he could to make life easier for them. Regency West was not a large apartment complex, but Edward and Daryl reserved five apartments for kidney patients. They charged very little and made the occupants as comfortable as possible. The location was fine, only a few blocks from the clinic.

It was necessary for them to sell the building after a short time, four years, to accommodate the need for expansion of the medical complex. The Methodist Hospital agreed with Edward's request that use of those five apartments would be continued for transplant patients until the building would be moved. It was comforting to know that some of its space would continue to be occupied by transplant patients.

In 1980 Edward bought the Brentwood Motor Inn Properties, a short distance from the clinic. He made this purchase with Daryl, Bob Sexton, whose wife, Sandy, had had a transplant two days after Edward's, and Fred Sexton, all of whom have been very close friends for more than twenty years. They offered substantial reduction in rates for kidney patients and their families. It was part of Edward's life to care for those with serious health problems. He knew very well that they had a desperate need for care beyond the clinical part.

One of Robert Kennedy's famous quotations is: "I dream of things that never were and say, 'Why not?' " Edward had such a dream. It was the beginning of his determination to find a place that could be a home away from home for transplant patients and their families. During this time, he was taking classes to earn the prestigious award: Certified Commercial Investment Member (CCIM). It was presented to him on November 16, 1981. He also received the Human Relations Award in 1988 from the Rochester Education Association with admiration and gratitude, and the J.C. Penny Golden Rule Lifetime Achievement Award in 1994.

His realty business gave him helpful knowledge about the availability of many properties. He wanted a house close to the Mayo Clinic with space for sleeping rooms, bathrooms, laundry, kitchen, and ample dining and family room quarters. He looked for a house that had been built when boarding homes were common, families were large, and motels were barely known.

Edward found his dream house at 624 West Center Street, the house that would become the Gift of Life Transplant House. He admits that he put the cart before the horse when he paid earnest money on it and made the commitment without funds and without an organization to operate the house. He just knew that with God's care this purchase would be finalized and that the patients could enjoy low-cost quarters and an opportunity to share with one another the good days and the bad. This home could be shared by, in addition to the kidney transplant patients, liver, bone-marrow, and heart transplant patients along with their families, and it has now expanded to include pancreas and lung patients.

Edward's enthusiasm and determination to actually buy the property helped him to organize a caring group of people to dedicate themselves to the enormous job that lay ahead. Amazingly, Edward himself raised the needed $15,000 for the required down payment. The money came from local businesses, a doctor, former patients, and others who believe they were investing in a truly humanitarian cause. A Rochester attorney and former transplant patient donated legal services, and Edward's accountant also provided services without charge. A number of hotels and motels volunteered furniture. Many people offered to clean, repair, paint, and give all other help as needed. Brentwood Motor Inn donated housekeeping services for a year, and the desk clerks there handled reservations until other arrangements could be made. Gifts of household items, linens, soaps, cleaning supplies, brooms, mops, paper towels, toilet tissue, etc., were bountiful and continued on through the years.

There was need to establish a system to determine which patients would be eligible to live at the Gift of Life Transplant House during their difficult times. It was decided that Social Services at the Mayo Clinic would inform such patients of the Gift of Life Transplant House and its charges of $5 to $10 per day. Social Services would then determine whose needs were valid for living there. Late in 1984 the house received its first guests.

Soon after the sale of Regency West, the name of Pompeian Engelhardt Realty was changed to Realty Growth, Inc. In the early days of the new business, Edward maintained his main office at the Brentwood. Some years later he moved the business to 1812 Second Street, Southwest, Rochester, where he remains at the current time.

Through the efforts of many people and the generosity of many organizations, businesses, and individuals the $100,000 mortgage on the Gift of Life Transplant House was retired on Monday, August 17, 1987, at a ceremony following a benefit celebrity golf tournament at the Rochester Country Club.

With the final payment made, the work soon began in the search for a much more spacious home to accommodate the ever-growing number of transplant patients.

There was no lessening of purpose and work among that group of dedicated people to find the future Gift of Life Transplant House. They were met by good fortune, and a very large, stately, and ideal home was found. This new home is perfect in structure (with renovation) and location, on the corner of Second Street and Seventh

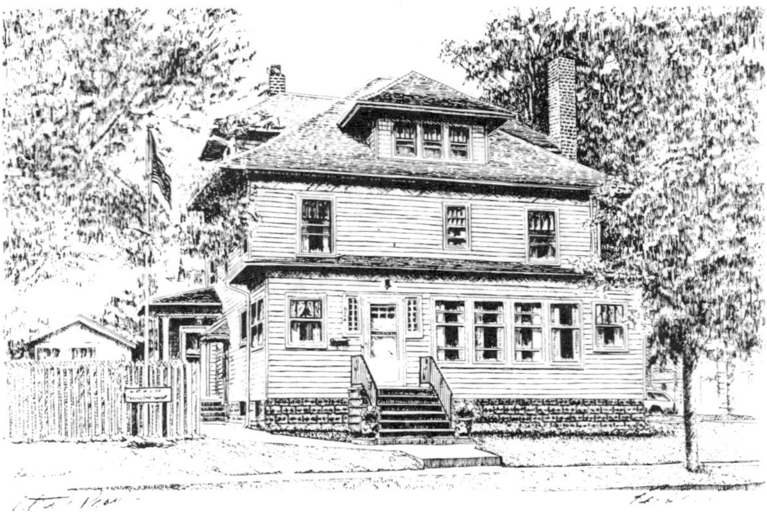

Gift of Life Transplant House   Founded 1984

Avenue, Southwest, only five blocks west from the Mayo Clinic. This home had been known for many years as the Judd House.

Dr. E. Starr Judd was a member of the original staff of the Mayo Clinic. Beginning in 1904 he became chief of the surgical staff. He was widely known and highly respected both in the United States and abroad.

The beautiful house was built for Dr. and Mrs. Judd in 1912. On July 10, 1931, for one dollar and other good and valuable consideration, Dr. and Mrs. Judd gave the property to the Mayo Foundation.

The Mayo Clinic Women's Club was given the use of it in 1938. In 1971 the club gave up its use, and the Intensive Psychotherapy Center was moved to the home from the Methodist Hospital.

Mrs. Eleanor Kirklin, a daughter of Dr. Judd, is deeply pleased that her old home will continue to have a humanitarian purpose in being a home away from home for many.

Epilogue

During the years of Edward's commitment to transplant patients and during his visits with them, he met and became friends with many other patients, physicians, nurses, technicians, and others. In Methodist Hospital at Station 54, the quarters for transplant patients, he was a familiar figure and a welcome guest.

In 1979 at Methodist Hospital while visiting a transplant patient friend, he met a nurse who later would become his wife. Edward was enchanted by her lovely smile and beautiful eyes. After several months of dating, the couple announced their engagement in April 1980.

Jayne Ann Diercks and Edward Paul Pompeian were married September 27, 1980, at Christ United Methodist Church in Rochester. Performing the candlelight ceremony was Rev. J. Charles Parker, a longtime friend and a transplant patient.

Jayne's matron of honor was her sister, Jean Lee, and the bridesmaids were Mary Rauterkus, Linda Usem, Candy Rustad, and Bobbie Jo Sexton. Edward's best man was Leon Sarkisian, my cousin, and the groomsmen were friends who also had successfully recovered from transplant surgery: Jim Bishop, David McMahon, and Larry Amundson. The others were my brother Richard, my grandson Paul, my nephew Nicky, and Jayne's cousin Greg. The soloist was Jennifer Woods and the organist was Julie Bjoraker.

At the wedding were many special guests, all of the doctors who had made it possible for Edward to receive

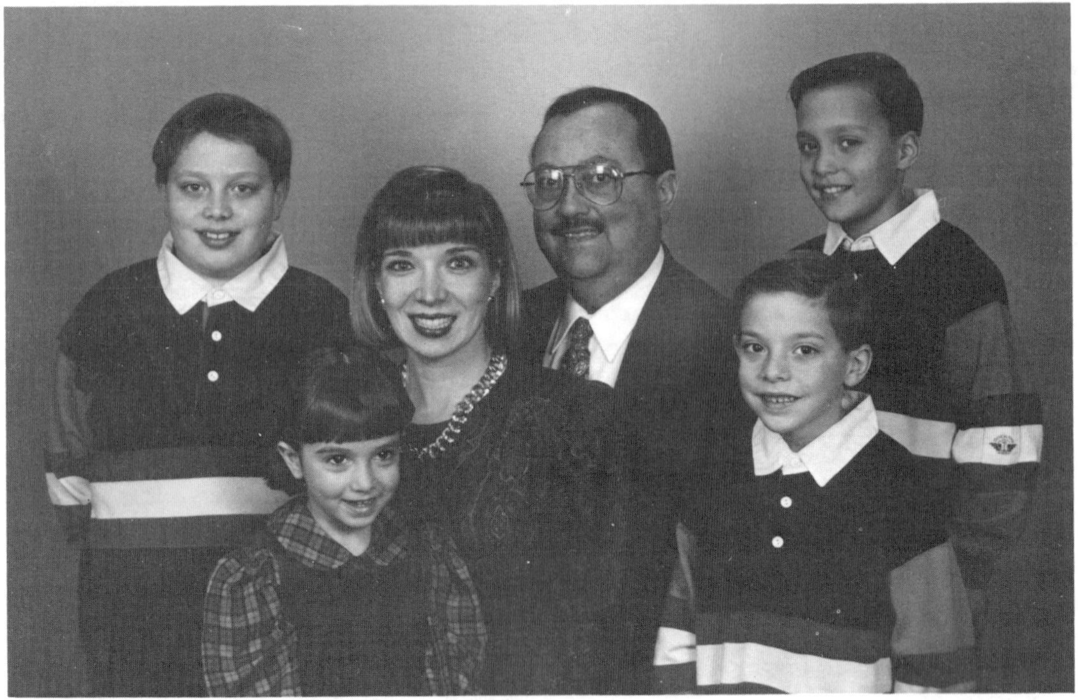

Edward and Jayne's family picture taken in November 1993. The children on the left are Edward and Adrienne; to the right are Aaron and Nicholas.

this great gift of life, members of both families, and many others.

Now, in 1995, Edward and Jayne have the joy of four talented children: Edward, Aaron, Nicholas, and Adrienne, from four to eleven years of age.

Edward continues to have an occasional health problem, and he continues the attitude and determination to "overcome." He always emerges successfully from these problems. His most recent need was for hip-joint replacement, which was performed in February 1994. He recovered remarkably well.

Edward's message is one of hope that more and more people will think seriously about filling out their donor cards and, in so doing, may one day make the difference in another person's life. He says, "Remember—organ and tissue donations make possible the God-given ability to give the gift of life."